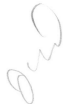

Monographs in Clinical Cytology

Vol. 26

Series Editor

Philippe Vielh Paris

Pancreatic Tumors

Volume Editors

Barbara A. Centeno Tampa, FL
Jasreman Dhillon Tampa, FL

107 figures, 100 in color, and 23 tables, 2020

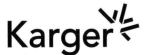

Basel · Freiburg · Hartford · Oxford · Bangkok · Dubai · Kuala Lumpur ·
Melbourne · Mexico City · Moscow · New Delhi · Paris · Shanghai · Tokyo

Monographs in Clinical Cytology

Founded 1965 by George L. Wied, Chicago, IL

Prof. Barbara A. Centeno
Department of Pathology
Moffitt Cancer Center
12902 USF Magnolia Drive
Tampa, FL 33612 (USA)
Barbara.Centeno@moffitt.org

Dr. Jasreman Dhillon
Associate Member and Associate Professor
Department of Pathology
Moffitt Cancer Center
12902 USF Magnolia Drive
Tampa, FL 33612 (USA)
Jasreman.Dhillon@moffitt.org

Library of Congress Cataloging-in-Publication Data

Names: Centeno, Barbara A., editor. | Dhillon, Jasreman, editor.
Title: Pancreatic tumors / volume editors, Barbara A. Centeno, Jasreman
 Dhillon.
Other titles: Pancreatic tumors (Centeno) | Monographs in clinical
 cytology ; v. 26. 0077-0809
Description: Basel ; Hartford : Karger, 2020. | Series: Monographs in
 clinical cytology, 0077-0809 ; vol. 26 | Includes bibliographical
 references and indexes. | Summary: "This book provides a comprehensive
 review of entities that may be encountered in pancreatic cytology. It is
 designed for cytotechnologists, pathology trainees, pathologists, and
 cytopathologists. It is also a useful guide for advanced endoscopists
 performing EUS-guided FNA, and surgeons and oncologists treating
 patients with pancreatic disease wanting to understand their pathology
 reports"-- Provided by publisher.
Identifiers: LCCN 2020022626 (print) | LCCN 2020022627 (ebook) | ISBN
 9783318066036 (hardcover ; alk. paper) | ISBN 9783318066043 (ebook)
Subjects: MESH: Pancreatic Neoplasms
Classification: LCC RC280.P25 (print) | LCC RC280.P25 (ebook) | NLM W1
 MO567KF v.26 2020 | DDC 616.99/437--dc23
LC record available at https://lccn.loc.gov/2020022626
LC ebook record available at https://lccn.loc.gov/2020022627

Bibliographic Indices. This publication is listed in bibliographic services, including Current Contents®.

© Copyright 2020 by S. Karger AG, P.O. Box, CH-4009 Basel (Switzerland)
www.karger.com
Printed on acid-free and non-aging paper (ISO 9706)
ISSN 0077–0809
ISBN 978–3–318–06603–6
e-ISBN 978–3–318–06604–3

Contents

Published online: September 29, 2020

Centeno BA, Dhillon J (eds): Pancreatic Tumors. Monogr Clin Cytol. Basel, Karger, 2020, vol 26, pp VI–VII (DOI:10.1159/000506356)

Preface

Image-guided fine-needle aspiration (FNA) of the pancreas using either transabdominal ultrasound or CT scan was first utilized and reported in the 1970s, eventually replacing laparotomy with wedge biopsy of the pancreas as the favored means of sampling pancreatic masses. In fact, this was the state of the field when the senior editor, Dr. Centeno was first introduced to pancreatic cytopathology as a first-year resident in 1988–1989. Endoscopic ultrasound (EUS)-guided FNA was first reported in 1992 as a means of guiding pancreatic aspiration. Initially received with some skepticism, it is now the preferred method used to perform FNA of the pancreas in many institutions throughout the world. The specific imaging features of many pancreatic lesions, using CT scan, transabdominal ultrasound, EUS, and now more advanced methods, such as magnetic resonance imaging and magnetic resonance cholangiopancreatography, have been described in detail.

Early publications on the cytology of the pancreas described the cytological features of ductal adenocarcinoma and its distinction from pancreatitis. As experience increased, the 1980s and 1990s saw numerous publications describing the cytological features of non-ductal neoplasms, as well as uncommon entities such as solid pseudopapillary neoplasm, formerly known as Frantz tumor, and pancreatoblastoma. A robust body of work also led to the develop-

ment of increasingly specific criteria for the challenging diagnosis of pancreatic ductal adenocarcinoma. Pancreatic cyst cytology was the next frontier of pancreatic cytology to be explored in the 1990s. In fact, the senior editor's first project in pancreatic cytopathology – started in her fellowship year in cytopathology – was to describe the cytological features of pancreatic cyst aspirates, derived from resection specimens. The recognition of the distinction of mucinous from non-mucinous lesions using cytology and measuring CEA cyst fluid levels was the next advance. FNA of pancreatic cysts is now accepted as part of the management protocol of patients with pancreatic cysts.

Yet, despite improved understanding of the cytological features of many entities, there remained challenging entities for which sensitivity of cytopathology is variable. More recently, evolution of the understanding of the genetics of pancreatic neoplasms has led to the development of immunohistochemical antibodies and molecular panels that provide more specific diagnoses and prognoses.

Pancreatic cytology is best practiced in a multidisciplinary manner. Accurate interpretation of the pancreatic cytology sample requires correlation of the clinical, imaging, cytological, and ancillary test findings. This volume provides the reader with the information necessary to assess a cytological specimen of the pancreas using a multidisciplinary approach. It describes and illustrates the cytological criteria of the most common non-neoplastic, neoplastic, and cystic lesions of the pancreas, and includes the pertinent clinical, imaging, and ancillary testing. A solid understanding of the histopathology of pancreatic lesions is also required to better evaluate pancreatic cytology. The histological features are included, and an approach to the differential diagnoses and potential pitfalls is reviewed.

This book provides a comprehensive review of entities that may be encountered in pancreatic cytology. It is designed for cytotechnologists, pathology trainees, pathologists, and cytopathologists. It is also a useful guide for advanced endoscopists performing EUS-guided FNA, and surgeons and oncologists treating patients with pancreatic disease wanting to understand their pathology reports.

The work presented here is the product of years of experience and curiosity of the senior editor, Dr. Centeno, who has witnessed the evolving landscape of pancreatic cytology, since the inception of EUS-guided FNA and pancreatic cyst fluid cytology. Dr. Centeno is honored to share her experience with the reader and to educate and mentor, with her colleague, Dr. Dhillon, the next generation of cytopathologists.

Barbara A. Centeno, Tampa, FL
Jasreman Dhillon, Tampa, FL

Chapter 1

Published online: September 29, 2020

Centeno BA, Dhillon J (eds): Pancreatic Tumors. Monogr Clin Cytol. Basel, Karger, 2020, vol 26, pp 1–14 (DOI:10.1159/000455729)

Introduction to Pancreatic Pathology and Fine-Needle Aspiration Cytology

Jasreman Dhillon[a, b]

[a]Department of Anatomic Pathology, Moffitt Cancer Center, Tampa, FL, USA; [b]Department of Oncologic Sciences and Pathology, University of South Florida, Tampa, FL, USA

Abstract

This introductory chapter discusses the demographics of pancreatic tumors and the risk factors associated with pancreatic neoplasms. The WHO 2019 classification of pancreatic epithelial tumors and WHO 2017 classification of pancreatic neuroendocrine neoplasms is provided. The current role of fine-needle aspiration (FNA) in the pancreatic lesions, different radiographic modalities and their evolution in the FNA of pancreatic lesions, and utility of rapid on-site evaluation of pancreatic cytology is also discussed. Guidelines on pancreatic pathology provided by the Papanicolaou Society of Cytopathology (PSC) in 2014 are summarized. These guidelines, which are provided by experts in the field, establish recommendations for clinical follow-up, indications, and preprocedural studies for pancreatic FNA, different techniques of pancreatic FNA, postprocedural follow-up, treatment options for different pancreatobiliary lesions, and utilization of ancillary studies for cytological diagnosis of pancreatic lesions. Standardization of the terminology and nomenclature and the diagnostic categories provided by the PSC are also discussed. Lastly, an algorithmic approach to cytological evaluation of pancreatic masses is provided.   © 2020 S. Karger AG, Basel

Demographics of Pancreatic Tumors

Primary malignant epithelial neoplasms of the pancreas are currently classified based on their phenotype into ductal, acinar, or neuroendocrine. Some remain unclassified as to their phenotype. Pancreatic ductal adenocarcinoma (PDAC) is the most common type, accounting for approximately 90% of the tumors [1].

Pancreatic cancer is the seventh leading cause of cancer deaths in the industrialized world and third most common in the USA [2]. Based on GLOBOCAN 18 estimates, it ranks as the eleventh most common cancer in the world, accounting for 4.5% of all deaths caused by cancer [2]. The highest mortality rates are in Western Europe (7.6 per 100,000 people), Central and Eastern Europe (7.3), and Northern Europe and North America equally (6.5). The lowest are in Eastern Africa (1.4) and South Eastern Asia and West Africa (2.1). Pancreatic cancer is trending to increase from 2018 to 2040 worldwide (+77.7% new cases and +79.9% deaths) [2].

The average lifetime risk of pancreatic cancer for both men and women is about 1 in 64 (1.6%). According to the American Cancer Society, about 57,600 people (30,400 men and 27,200 women) will be diagnosed with pancreatic cancer in the year 2020 and about 47,050 people will die of pancreatic cancer in the USA (www.cancer.org).

Table 1. Syndromes and their associated gene mutations

a Syndromes and their associated gene mutations that are known to increase the risk of developing pancreatic adenocarcinoma

Predisposition syndromes	Genes
Familial breast cancer	ATM, PALB2
Hereditary breast and ovarian cancer	BRCA1, BRCA2
Familial atypical mole and melanoma	CDKN2A
Hereditary non-polyposis colorectal cancer (Lynch syndrome)	Mismatch repair: MLH1, MSH2, MSH6, PMS2
Hereditary pancreatitis	PRSS1, SPINK2
Peutz-Jeghers syndrome	STK11
Ataxia telangiectasia	ATM

b Syndromes and their associated gene mutations that are known to increase the risk of developing pancreatic neuroendocrine tumors

Syndrome	Gene mutated
MEN1	MEN1
Tuberous sclerosis	TSC1, TSC2
VHL	VHL
Neurofibromatosis type 1	NF1

The incidence increases with age for both sexes [2]. Pancreatic cancer is usually present in patients older than 65 years of age, with a median age at diagnosis of 71 years. There is a slight preponderance in men. Risk factors associated with pancreatic cancer include older age, smoking, obesity, and exposure to certain chemicals used in dry cleaning and metal industries. Smoking is a firmly established risk factor for pancreatic cancer [3]. Compared to those who have never smoked, the overall risk is 1.40 for ever cigarette smokers, 1.17 for former cigarette smokers, and 2.2 for current cigarette smokers [3]. The risk of PDAC decreases with smoking cessation. Another potentially modifiable factor implicated in the development of pancreas cancer is a high body mass index (BMI). Insulin resistance is hypothesized as a mechanism contributing to this increase in risk in patients with a high BMI [4].

A family history of pancreatic cancer, usually defined as having at least one affected first degree relative, is seen in 5–10% of individuals with this disease [5, 6]. Risk is known to increase strongly in families with several members affected [7]. Familial pancreatic cancer characterizes families with an abnormally high rate of pancreatic cancer in which an inherited gene is suspected but has not been identified. Individuals with familial pancreatic cancer may have a spe-

cific genetic mutation that is linked to a syndrome which predisposes them to certain types of cancer. Mutations in a number of genes are related to increased risk of PDAC. Currently, at least twelve inherited gene mutations are known to increase the predisposition to pancreatic cancer [8]. The genetic syndromes included are hereditary breast and ovarian cancer syndrome, familial atypical multiple mole melanoma syndrome, familial pancreatitis, Lynch syndrome, and Peutz-Jeghers syndrome. *PALB2* and *ATM* have recently been associated with familial cancers [8]. The inherited syndromes and gene mutations associated with pancreatic cancer are shown in Table 1a.

Other neoplasms and malignancies are less common. Pancreatic neuroendocrine tumors (PanNETs) comprise approximately 5% of pancreatic malignant tumors [1] and occur sporadically. PanNETs are rarely seen in children and adolescents, but when present are usually associated with a genetic/familial [9] predisposition such as multiple endocrine neoplasia 1 (MEN1), tuberous sclerosis, von Hippel-Lindau (VHL) disease, and neurofibromatosis (Table 1b). Acinar cell carcinoma (ACC) is a rare malignant neoplasm, comprising 1–2% of pancreatic malignant tumors with a mean age of presentation of 56 years [1]. Approximately 6% of ACCs occur in children between the ages of 8 and 15 years

[1]. The clinical evolution of this neoplasm in children seems to be better than that observed in adults [10]. Pancreatoblastoma is a rare tumor comprising <1% of malignant pancreatic tumors that is said to have a bimodal peak first at 5 years and then at 40 years of age [1]. Solid-pseudopapillary neoplasm (SPN) comprises 1–2% of the pancreatic tumors [1] and occurs predominantly in young females.

Pancreatic Tumor Classification

The 2019 World Health Organization (WHO) classifies pancreatic tumors into epithelial tumors, mature teratoma, mesenchymal tumors, lymphomas, and secondary tumors that are defined as neoplasms that have spread to the pancreas from an extra-pancreatic primary. The WHO 2019 classification of pancreatic epithelial tumors is provided in Table 2a, and the WHO 2017 classification of pancreatic neuroendocrine neoplasms, incorporated into the WHO 2019 classification of digestive system tumors [1], is provided in Table 2b.

History and Current Concepts of Fine-Needle Aspiration Cytology of Pancreatic Tumors

Before the advent of endoscopic ultrasonography (EUS), percutaneous ultrasonography (US)-guided fine-needle aspiration (FNA) biopsies and computed tomography (CT)-guided FNA biopsies were utilized for obtaining tissue for cytological examination. Beginning in the 1970s, US was the first imaging modality used, with the use of CT reported a few years later [11, 12]. EUS was developed in the 1980s to overcome limitations of transabdominal US imaging of the pancreas caused by intervening gas, bone, and fat, and is currently the most common source of obtaining material from pancreatic lesions. EUS provides excellent visualization of the pancreatic head and uncinate process from the duodenum as well as the body and tail of the pancreas from the stomach. With the advent of curvilinear echo endoscopes, both transgastric and transduodenal EUS-guided FNA (EUS-FNA) biopsies of the pancreas have become a possibility. EUS is superior to percutaneous US and CT scan, especially when the pancreatic tumor is <2–3 cm [13, 14]. In hospitals where CT-guided biopsies and/or endoscopic retrograde cholangiopancreatography (ERCP) brushings are still the standard methods for obtaining tissue for diagnosis of pancreatic lesions, false negative rates of

>30% have been reported [15]. Advantages of EUS-FNA over other modalities include the close proximity of the target lesion to the endoscope, sampling under direct ultrasound guidance, and avoidance of overlying bowel [16].

Accuracy of FNA in Pancreatic Tumors
The reported diagnostic yield of EUS-FNA for pancreatic tumorous lesions is good, with a diagnostic accuracy of 78–95%, sensitivity of 78–95%, and specificity of 75–100% [17–19]. EUS-FNA has a high specificity but a low sensitivity for diagnosing malignancy in pancreatic cystic tumors.

False positive and false negative rates of cytological diagnosis of pancreatic masses on EUS-FNA are low. The false positive rate is about 2% and results from technical difficulties and sampling or interpretation errors. False positive results due to interpretation errors can occur from contamination of the specimen by an intervening mucosal malignancy, or misinterpretation of reactive changes in chronic pancreatitis as adenocarcinoma [20]. Chronic pancreatitis is the most common benign pathology causing false positive interpretation of a pancreatic cancer.

Rapid On-Site Evaluation
Rapid on-site evaluation (ROSE) performed by the cytopathologist at the time of an endoscopic procedure is necessary to direct the endosonographer as to whether the aspirate obtained is sufficient for a definitive diagnosis. This not only means that there is enough diagnostic material in the smears, but also that there is sufficient material for an ancillary work-up. The direct smears obtained in the endoscopy suite are quickly processed and examined by a light microscope and immediate direct feedback is provided to the endosonographer. This information assists in guiding the endosonographer to the number of EUS-FNA passes required and whether the biopsy technique needs to be adjusted in non-diagnostic aspirates to yield material for a final diagnosis. ROSE is generally performed on solid pancreatic masses and not on cystic pancreatic lesions. Non-ROSE groups were shown to have more repeat EUS-FNA biopsies than ROSE groups and this difference was reported to be statistically significant in some studies [21]. However, many recent studies have reported adequacy rates of pancreatic FNA to be similar with and without ROSE, indicating that, perhaps, at high-volume centres and in expert hands, ROSE may not be indispensable to achieve excellent results [22–24]. Up to four passes are usually recommended to get diagnostic material for pancreatic FNAs as it has been shown that the chances of aspirating diagnostic material decrease after that

Table 2. WHO classifications

a WHO 2019 classification of epithelial tumors (excluding pancreatic neuroendocrine neoplasms) of the pancreas [1]

Category	Tumor/lesion type

Benign epithelial tumors and precursors	Serous cystadenoma not otherwise specified (NOS)
	    Macrocystic (oligocystic) serous cystadenoma
	    Solid serous adenoma
	    VHL syndrome-associated serous cystic neoplasm
	    Mixed serous-neuroendocrine neoplasm
	Serous cystadenocarcinoma NOS
	Glandular intraepithelial neoplasia, low grade
	Glandular intraepithelial neoplasia, high grade
	Intraductal papillary mucinous neoplasm with low-grade dysplasia
	Intraductal papillary mucinous neoplasm with high-grade dysplasia
	Intraductal papillary mucinous neoplasm with associated invasive carcinoma
	Intraductal oncocytic papillary neoplasm NOS
	Intraductal oncocytic papillary neoplasm with associated invasive carcinoma
	Intraductal tubulopapillary neoplasm
	Intraductal tubulopapillary neoplasm with associated invasive carcinoma
	Mucinous cystic neoplasm with low-grade dysplasia
	Mucinous cystic neoplasm with high-grade dysplasia
	Mucinous cystic neoplasm with associated invasive carcinoma

Malignant epithelial tumors	Ductal adenocarcinoma NOS
	    Adenosquamous carcinoma
	    Colloid carcinoma (mucinous non-cystic carcinoma)
	    Hepatoid carcinoma
	    Medullary carcinoma NOS
	    Signet-ring cell carcinoma
	    Carcinoma, undifferentiated, NOS
	    Undifferentiated carcinoma with osteoclast-like giant cells
	    Poorly cohesive carcinoma
	    Large-cell carcinoma with rhabdoid phenotype
	Carcinomas with acinar differentiation
	    Acinar cell carcinoma
	    Acinar cell cystadenocarcinoma
	    Mixed acinar-neuroendocrine carcinoma
	    Mixed acinar-endocrine-ductal carcinoma
	    Mixed acinar-ductal carcinoma
	Solid-pseudopapillary neoplasm
	    Solid pseudopapillary neoplasm with high-grade carcinoma
	Pancreatoblastoma

b WHO 2017 classification and grading of pancreatic neuroendocrine neoplasms (PanNENs) [1]

Classification/grade	Ki-67 proliferation index	Mitotic index
Well-differentiated PanNENs: PanNETs		
PanNET G1	<3%	<2
PanNET G2	3–20%	2–20
PanNET G3	>20%	>20
Poorly differentiated PanNETs: pancreatic neuroendocrine carcinomas (PanNECs)		
PanNEC (G3)	>20%	>20
Small cell neuroendocrine carcinoma		
Large cell neuroendocrine carcinoma		
Mixed neuroendocrine-non-neuroendocrine neoplasm		

[25, 26]. However, certain solid neoplasms of the pancreas are desmoplastic and hence may provide few cells that could be insufficient to provide a definitive diagnosis. ROSE is particularly helpful in these cases so that more aspirates can be obtained to increase the yield for a definitive diagnosis and to ensure that the patient does not have to undergo a repeat FNA at a later date.

Papanicolaou Society of Cytopathology Guidelines for Pancreatobiliary Cytology

Summary of the Guidelines

The Papanicolaou Society of Cytopathology (PSC) developed a set of guidelines for pancreatobiliary cytology similar to those developed for other organ systems, which assess indications and techniques for imaging and FNA, terminology and nomenclature of pancreatobiliary disease, and available ancillary testing and post-biopsy management. These were published and summarized in 2014 [27–31]. These guidelines were developed based on the authors' expertise, review of the literature, discussion of the draft documents at national and international meetings, and synthesis of online comments of the draft documents. The subsequent sections summarize the recommendations of the PSC in each topic, focused on pancreatic disease.

Recommendations for Clinical Evaluation, Imaging Studies, Indications for Cytologic Study, and Preprocedural Requirements for Pancreatic FNA

The PSC has proposed recommendations for clinical evaluation, imaging studies, indications for cytological study, and preprocedural requirements for pancreatic FNA [27]. The clinical presentation of pancreatic neoplasia may include newly diagnosed late-onset diabetes mellitus, unexplained pancreatitis in an older individual, development of obstructive jaundice, pruritus, cholestasis, abdominal pain that radiates to the back, anorexia, weight loss, and steatorrhea. Elevated liver enzymes or imaging studies may indicate the presence of metastatic disease and confirm the presence of malignancy.

According to the PSC recommendations, patients with suspected pancreatic neoplasm should receive the following [27]:

1. A thorough history and physical examination. The history should include assessment for risk factors for the development of pancreatic adenocarcinoma, possible familial cancer history, and history of previous

malignancy. The history should also include an assessment of risk factors for benign conditions such as pancreatitis.
2. Laboratory studies to assess bilirubin and alkaline phosphatase, and serum tumor markers, carbonic anhydrase (CA19-9), and carcinoembryonic antigen (CEA) should be conducted.
3. All of these patients should undergo imaging studies.
4. Benign conditions such as chronic pancreatitis, primary sclerosing cholangitis, and autoimmune diseases should be excluded. A serum IgG4 would be beneficial to exclude IgG4-related disease.

A number of imaging modalities may be used when assessing patients with clinically suspected pancreatic neoplasia. These include transabdominal US, CT, EUS, magnetic resonance imaging (MRI), magnetic resonance angiography, and magnetic resonance cholangiopancreatography. The indications and utility of these imaging studies will be discussed in detail in the chapter by Morse and Klapman [this vol., pp. 21–33].

The imaging work-up of solid masses is usually performed to determine if the mass is benign or malignant, or possibly of some other morphology. If malignant, the work-up is focused on determining resectability, as described by Morse and Klapman [this vol., pp. 23–28]. Patients with evidence of resectable solid pancreatic masses may be referred directly to surgery without a prior FNA, but this approach is not advocated because of the risk of unusual morphologies. A definitive diagnosis is needed for patients who are not surgical candidates or who need to have neoadjuvant therapy, which is increasingly being used for borderline resectable cases, and FNA is the preferred sampling method in this group of patients.

The work-up of pancreatic cysts is focused on determining if the cyst is mucinous (premalignant) or non-mucinous (serous, developmental, or inflammatory). Pancreatic cysts are usually first evaluated by CT scan. ERCP and EUS can be used for further evaluation. The 2012 international consensus guidelines for the management of intraductal papillary mucinous neoplasm (IPMN) and mucinous cystic neoplasm (MCN) of the pancreas, and more recent 2017 revisions to the international consensus Fukuoka guidelines, attempt to standardize the work-up and management of patients with neoplastic mucinous cysts [32] and IPMN [33]. The 2017 guidelines are provided in Figure 1. Briefly, depending upon the size of the mucinous cyst, follow-up and treatment options may differ. Conservative management is recommended for mucinous cysts <3 cm in the absence of

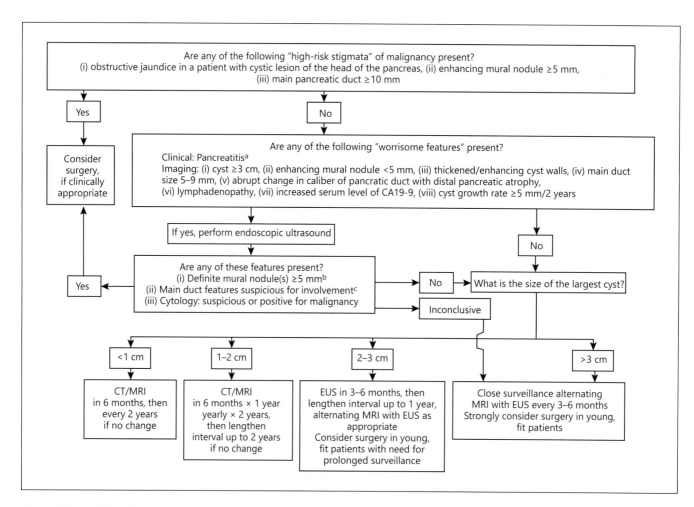

Fig. 1. 2017 revisions of international consensus Fukuoka guidelines for the management of IPMN of the pancreas. Algorithm for the management of suspected BD-IPMN. [a]Pancreatitis may be an indication for surgery for relief of symptoms. [b]Differential diagnosis includes mucin. Mucin can move with change in patient position, may be dislodged on cyst lavage and does not have Doppler flow. Features of true tumor nodule include lack of mobility, presence of Doppler flow and FNA of nodule showing tumor tissue. [c]Presence of any one of thickened walls, intraductal mucin or mural nodules is suggestive of main duct involvement. In their absence main duct involvement is inconclusive. Abbreviations: BD-IPMN, branch duct intraductal papillary mucinous neoplasm; FNA, fine needle aspiration. Reproduced from Tanaka et al. [33] with permission from Elsevier.

high-risk clinical and radiographic findings. High-risk radiographic findings include a solid enhancing lesion within the cyst or a main pancreatic duct ≥10 mm in diameter. High-risk clinical findings include obstructive jaundice and a cystic lesion in the head of the pancreas. Worrisome features include a cyst 3 cm or more in size, enhancing mural nodule <5 mm, thickened/enhancing cyst wall, main pancreatic duct diameter 5–9 mm, a non-enhancing mural nodule, an abrupt change in the caliber of the main pancreatic duct with distal pancreatic atrophy, lymphadenopathy, increased serum level of CA19-9, and cyst growth rate ≥5 mm/2 years [27, 33]. In the absence of high-risk and worri-

some features, cysts <1 cm are followed by MRI/CT scans in 6 months and then every 2 years if there is no change; cysts of 1–2 or 2–3 cm are followed by MRI/CT scans in 6 months and then every year for 2 years if there is no change, or 6 months for a year and then yearly, respectively. For young patients with a 2- to 3-cm cyst without worrisome features with prolonged surveillance, surgery should be considered.

EUS, when available, should be used for preoperative staging in patients with suspected pancreatic carcinoma or cancer of the biliary tract. It is particularly useful when CT or MRI findings are equivocal. EUS appears to be superior for detecting small masses, evaluating for tumor involvement of the superior mesenteric vein and the portal vein, and detecting lymph node metastases [34–36].

Pre-FNA requirements include obtaining informed consent. An informed consent form has to be signed by a competent patient before pancreatic FNA is performed. The possibility of complications such as bleeding, allergic/cardiac/respiratory reaction, and/or perforation should be mentioned in the consent form. An informed consent form should also include an explanation of the FNA procedure and inform patients that the results of the procedure may be non-contributory.

Techniques for Cytological Sampling of Pancreatic Lesions
The PSC published guidelines for sampling of pancreatobiliary lesions. This section will focus only on FNA of pancreatic masses. ERCP-guided brush cytology of the pancreatic duct can be performed for sampling of the main pancreatic duct in which a wire-guided brush is used to collect cells from a strictured pancreatic duct.

A number of imaging modalities may be used to guide pancreatic FNA, including US, EUS, and CT scans. EUS FNA is now the procedure of choice in establishing the diagnosis of a pancreatic lesion. Linear endosonographic instruments are required to target lesions for FNA [37]. Simple aspiration needles (usually 22- or 25-G) are used for the procedure. Both caliber needles yield the same cytologic material [38]. Smaller 25-G needles are preferable for sampling suspected PDAC as they are easier to use. They are also preferred for vascular lesions and aspiration of lymph nodes. Core biopsy and Tru-Cut needles are used for lesions such as stromal cell tumors, panNETs, and tumors with a suboptimal cytology yield and lesions suspicious for autoimmune pancreatitis. The EUS-FNA procedure can be difficult to perform due to vessel interposition, duodenal stenosis, bleeding, and tumor firmness. Prior gastric surgery or bypass will limit accessibility of the device to the pancreas. A 22-G beveled needle called Procore (Echo Tip) is available for use with the EUS device that produces a core-like tissue fragment.

Mucinous cysts are aspirated using a 22-G needle due to the high viscosity of the cyst fluid. Serous cystadenomas and cystic NETs should be aspirated with a 25-G needle as the cyst fluid is not viscous. Pseudocysts should be aspirated with a 22- or 19-G needle in order to evacuate the entire lesion, which may become contaminated by FNA. Mural nodules and any adjacent masses can be aspirated after the cyst fluid is aspirated. The cyst fluid is centrifuged and may be sent for CEA and DNA mutational analysis.

Standardized Terminology and Nomenclature
The PSC has developed a set of guidelines for the terminology and nomenclature of pancreatobiliary disease [28]. The proposed terminology recommends a six-tiered system comprising non-diagnostic, negative, atypical, neoplastic (benign and other), suspicious, and positive (Table 3).

Non-diagnostic specimens are those that provide no diagnostic or useful information. This may be due to technical or sampling issues. Absence of epithelial cells should not be presumed to be non-diagnostic as sampling from pancreatic pseudocysts and mucinous cysts can be acellular. Clinical and radiographic information is helpful in these instances. In the presence of any cellular atypia, the non-diagnostic category should not be used. Cytological interpretation can be limited by the amount of material aspirated or by preparation artifact such as tissue entrapped in a blood clot precluding cytological evaluation. The presence of only gastrointestinal contaminants or normal pancreatic tissue in the context of a well-defined pancreatic mass are some examples that should be included in this category.

A negative cytology is a sample that contains adequate tissue to define a lesion that is identified on radiology. It may indicate benign entities like acute, chronic, and autoimmune pancreatitis, pseudocyst, ectopic, and intrapancreatic splenule and lymphoepithelial cyst.

Atypical categories include cases with features that are more than reactive changes, low cellularity, premalignant (dysplastic) changes, and cases assigned due to observer caution. The cytological specimen may contain cells with morphological features beyond recognizable normal or reactive changes. An atypical diagnosis raises the possibility of a neoplasm, especially a low-grade neoplasm. The "neoplastic" category is separated into "benign," which includes neoplasms such as serous cystadenoma, and "other," which includes premalignant lesions such as mucinous cysts, IPMN, and low-grade malignant tumors such as PanNETs and SPN.

The PSC guidelines use the term "suspicious for malignancy" to cover a range of atypias falling just short of that necessary for a definitive diagnosis of malignancy. These specimens lack sufficient diagnostic features for a definitive diagnosis. Other information, such as clinical, imaging, or ancillary test findings, must be correlated with the cytologic findings before surgical intervention can be undertaken.

The positive category includes malignant neoplasms such as PDAC, ACC, poorly differentiated neuroendocrine carcinomas, pancreatoblastoma, lymphoma, and metasta-

Table 3. Standardized terminology for pancreatic cytology by the PSC

Diagnostic category	Definition
Non-diagnostic	Specimen that provides no diagnostic or useful information about the solid or cystic lesion samples
Negative (for malignancy)	Specimen that contains adequate cellular and extracellular to define a lesion identified on imaging (acute or chronic pancreatitis, autoimmune pancreatitis, pseudocyst, lymphoepithelial cyst, splenule/accessory spleen)
Atypical	Cells present with cytoplasmic, nuclear, or architectural features that are not consistent with normal or reactive cellular changes of the pancreas or bile ducts and are insufficient to classify them as a neoplasm or suspicious for a high-grade malignancy; the findings are insufficient to establish an abnormality explaining the lesion seen on imaging; follow-up evaluation is warranted
Neoplastic: benign or other	*Neoplastic: benign* Cytological specimen that is diagnostic of a benign neoplasm such as IPMN or MCN with dysplasia (low/intermediate/high grade) *Neoplastic: other* Neoplasm that is either premalignant or is a low-grade malignant neoplasm (PanNET, SPN)
Suspicious (for malignancy)	The cytological features raise a strong suspicion for malignancy, but the findings are qualitatively and/or quantitatively insufficient for a conclusive diagnosis, or tissue is not present for ancillary studies to define a specific neoplasm
Positive/malignant	A group of neoplasms that unequivocally display malignant cytologic characteristics and include pancreatic ductal adenocarcinoma and its variants, cholangiocarcinoma, acinar cell carcinoma, high-grade neuroendocrine carcinoma (small cell and large cell), pancreatoblastoma, lymphomas, sarcomas, and metastases to the pancreas

PSC, Papanicolaou Society of Cytopathology; IPMN, intraductal papillary mucinous neoplasm; MCN, mucinous cystic neoplasm; PanNET, pancreatic neuroendocrine tumor; SPN, solid pseudopapillary neoplasm.

ses. This category is used when unequivocal features of malignancy are identified.

FNA Biopsy Follow-Up and Treatment Options for Patients with Pancreatobiliary Lesions
This work group focused on developing management recommendations based on the proposed terminology [30]. This section summarizes those recommendations.

Recommendations based on the recommended diagnostic categories are as follows:

Non-Diagnostic
The PSC recommends a repeat FNA procedure when the first attempt yields a non-diagnostic cytology sample. The clinical team may elect to proceed to laparotomy without repetition depending on the radiographic and clinical findings for obtaining a Tru-Cut needle biopsy. If the first attempt was via brushings, it can be repeated by brushings or EUS-FNA. If the first attempt was by percutaneous FNA then it may be most reasonable to use EUS-FNA for the second attempt. If the first attempt was EUS-FNA, reassessment of the EUS findings and other imaging should be undertaken, followed by a review of the FNA line of approach [30]. Repeat aspiration of a cystic lesion of the pancreas should be carefully considered due to there being up to 14% risk of associated infection.

Negative
A negative cytology may indicate benign entities like acute, chronic, and autoimmune pancreatitis, pseudocyst, ectopic

and intrapancreatic splenule, and lymphoepithelial cyst. If cytopathology is diagnostic of a specific benign entity, then the treatment is aimed to treat that particular entity. However, if the negative cytology diagnosis is descriptive without a specific benign entity diagnosis, it should not be taken to be synonymous with a benign lesion. The multidisciplinary team should evaluate the clinical presentation, radiographic findings, and cytopathology, and should reassess the component that is discrepant. False negative interpretations are not uncommon in pancreatic EUS-FNA due to sampling and interpretive errors. If the lesion is clinically suspicious, FNA may be repeated to collect diagnostic material.

Atypical

Cytologic specimens categorized as atypical demonstrate cytologic and architectural alterations that are greater than reactive atypia, but less than that of suspicious for malignancy. It is not trivial to repeat pancreatic FNAs diagnosed as atypical as there are a number of individuals involved and use of expensive equipment makes the resource utilization and costs of operative biopsy even greater. The appropriate course of action is dependent on a multidisciplinary review, the functional status of the patient, and the wishes of the patient after clinical consultation [30]. An atypical interpretation on cytology may require additional diagnostic tests such as loss of immunohistochemical staining for the *Dpc4/SMAD4* suppressor gene and detection of mutant *KRAS* that may contribute to management decisions when imaging is suspicious for adenocarcinoma. Ancillary tests such as fluorescent in situ hybridization (FISH) and next-generation sequencing have shown promise in improving diagnostic sensitivity for the detection of malignancy [39, 40]. The related malignancy risk of the atypical category for EUS-FNAs of solid pancreatic masses is 25–100% (mean 58%) [41–43].

Neoplastic: Benign

The major lesion in this category is serous cystic neoplasm (SCN), which can either be observed or treated by resection. If imaging, cytology, and cyst fluid biochemistry (CEA and amylase) support an interpretation of an SCN, the patient can be conservatively managed with observation. However, if the patient is symptomatic and there is evidence of significant growth, which increases the risk of hemorrhage and rupture, it is resected.

Neoplastic: Other

Pancreatic Neuroendocrine Tumor. PanNETs can either be managed conservatively by observation or by surgery, depending upon the clinical scenario. Very small (close to 1 cm), incidentally discovered PanNETs in elderly patients with multiple comorbid conditions may be managed conservatively. PanNETs may grow very slowly for prolonged periods. Although the majority (50–60%) exhibit malignant behavior, surgical intervention may not be the best option, especially for elderly patients with multiple comorbidities. Hence, PSC has placed PanNETs in the "neoplastic: other" rather than in the "malignant" category so that patients can have more conservative management options as well. Genetic testing for germline mutations may be performed in cases where family or personal history is suggestive of MEN1 or VHL disease. Medical management of functioning PanNETs is available with multiple drugs, especially in non-resectable cases. For patients with metastatic disease, if the disease is restricted to the liver, resection (including the possibility of hepatectomy and transplantation) is warranted for both functioning and non-functioning tumors with the aim of curative resection or debulking/palliative treatment depending on the size and location of the tumor [30]. Radiofrequency ablation or embolization may be considered with or without chemotherapy for liver metastases.

Solid-Pseudopapillary Neoplasm. Surgical resection is the treatment of choice for SPN.

Mucinous Cystic Neoplasm. MCNs are mostly benign, with 18% of cases undergoing malignant transformation. Hence, due to the expense and anxiety associated with life-long surveillance, these neoplasms are removed surgically regardless of their grade. However, patients with small cysts and without high-risk imaging features can be managed with observation.

Intraductal Papillary Mucinous Neoplasms. IPMNs are treated with either surgical resection or observation depending upon the location. IPMNs that involve the main pancreatic duct are treated with resection. IPMNs that involve only branch ducts can be treated by either of the two options. The decision to operate depends upon the presence of worrisome imaging features such as a large cyst size (>3 cm) or a non-enhancing mural nodule. IPMNs with cytological presence of high-grade dysplasia and adenocarcinoma are surgically resected. Figure 1 shows the Fukuoka revised guidelines for the management of MCNs and IPMNs.

Gastrointestinal Stromal Tumor. Surgical resection is the treatment of choice for localized gastrointestinal stromal tumors (GISTs). For advanced or metastatic c-Kit-positive GISTs, tyrosine kinase inhibitor (TKI) imatinib is used. Patients who develop resistance to TKI are treated with chemotherapy.

Suspicious

Suspicious findings on cytology are generally correlated with the clinical and imaging findings, and if radiology favors a malignant neoplasm the patient may be worked up and staged. Biochemical and molecular analytical markers may increase the sensitivity and specificity of the interpretation [26]. If the cytological findings are suspicious whereas imaging findings are benign, then a repeat sampling of the lesion should be considered.

Positive/Malignant

Adenocarcinoma of the Pancreas. For adenocarcinomas of the pancreas, if resectable, surgery is the initial option (Whipple's procedure for tumors in the head or uncinate process and distal pancreatectomy and splenectomy for tumors in the body and tail) with adjuvant chemotherapy. In cases of non-resectable disease or metastatic disease patients are treated with chemotherapy.

Acinar Cell Carcinoma. Treatment of ACC is similar to that of PDAC.

High-Grade Neuroendocrine Carcinoma (Small Cell and Large Cell Type). These tumors are treated with chemotherapy regimens that are similar to small cell carcinomas of the lung [44].

Pancreatoblastoma. Surgical resection with adjuvant or neoadjuvant chemotherapy is the preferred treatment for pancreatoblastomas.

Lymphoma. Lymphomas are medically managed depending upon the specific type, including histologic morphology, flow cytometry, and cytogenetic findings.

Metastases. Diagnosis of metastasis generally indicates a widespread malignancy that is managed according to its specific subtype.

For further details, strategies provided by surgical and gastrointestinal specialty organizations, including the British Society of Gastroenterology, the Pancreatic Society of Great Britain, the Royal College of Pathology, the Japan Pancreas Society, the International Association of Pancreatology [45, 46], and the National Comprehensive Cancer Network (NCCN) [47], can be referred to.

Utilization of Ancillary Studies in the Cytologic Diagnosis of Pancreatic Lesions

Ancillary techniques that help in refining the cytological diagnosis are invaluable. A good cell block containing ample material is required. Ancillary tests include biochemical and molecular tests and immunohistochemical and special stains. These tests have diagnostic and prognostic implications. The PSC made recommendations on the utilization of ancillary studies [29]. These are further expanded upon in subsequent chapters of this monograph. Indications for ancillary testing in the pancreas include the following scenarios: differentiation of benign from malignant ductal lesions, diagnosis of primary and metastatic neoplasms, work-up of suspected hematopoietic lesions, and preoperative work-up of pancreatic cysts.

Several studies have found *KRAS* mutations in the premalignant dysplastic lesions and invasive carcinomas of the pancreas [48–53]. Although *KRAS* mutation analysis is a sensitive test for pancreatic adenocarcinoma, it can also test positive in benign cases such as chronic pancreatitis [50, 51]. Current data do not support *KRAS* testing in solid pancreatic masses. The PSC recommends the use of commercially available UroVysion FISH testing (Abbott Molecular, Abbott Park, IL, USA) on brushings from pancreatobiliary strictures with cytological diagnosis of indeterminate atypia. This test analyzes individual cells for DNA abnormality to determine if the sample is positive or negative. FISH analysis outperforms routine cytology with very high specificity and much higher sensitivity for the identification of carcinoma [54–56].

For the assessment of pancreatic cystic lesions, ancillary tests that aid in the diagnosis are CA19-9, CEA, and amylase levels in the cyst fluid, and some special stains. Special stains such as periodic acid-Schiff (PAS) and PAS with diastase (dPAS) detect the presence of glycogen. Glycogen is present in the clear cytoplasm of the cuboidal cells of serous cystadenoma and in the zymogen granules of the acinar cell lesions. PAS, mucicarmine (for neutral mucin), and Alcian blue (acid mucin) are used to detect the presence of intracellular and extracellular mucin. The cyst fluid CEA level is a very good test to diagnose if the cyst is mucinous, in which case the level usually exceeds 192 ng/mL [57]. Cyst fluid amylase levels help to diagnose pseudocyst where the levels are typically elevated into thousands. This test, however, does not distinguish IPMN from MCN as both can show slightly elevated levels.

Immunostaining for Smad4 is a good surrogate for *SMAD4* genetic alterations and is useful in establishing a diagnosis of adenocarcinoma as it is retained in benign pancreatic ducts and is lost in more than half of PDACs [58]. Overexpression of mesothelin favors a diagnosis of adenocarcinoma. Trypsin and chymotrypsin positivity helps to diagnose ACC.

For PanNETs, immunostains synaptophysin, chromogranin, and the proliferation marker Ki-67 can be extremely

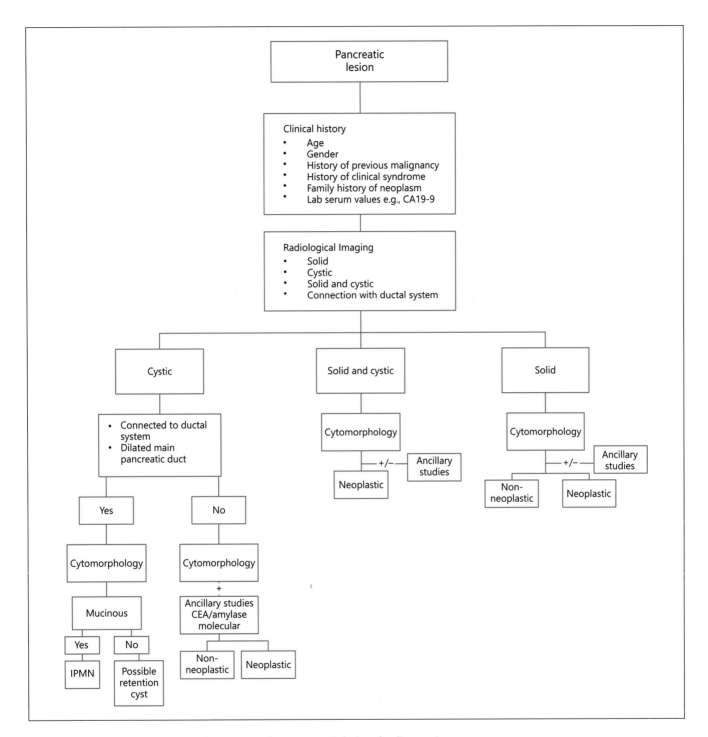

Fig. 2. Flowchart depicting an algorithmic approach to pancreatic lesions for diagnostic purposes.

helpful. Ki-67 is of importance in the histologic grading of PanNETs, but its utility in cytological preparations remains to be determined [59]. Strong nuclear staining for beta-catenin is diagnostic for SPNs in the pancreas.

Cystic lesions of the pancreas exhibit a specific distinctive mutational profile for each subtype. SCNs have *VHL* mutations, *CTNNB1* mutation is diagnostic of SPNs, MCNs have mutations involving the *RNF43, KRAS, TP53*, and *SMAD4* genes, and IPMNs have mutations involving the genes *KRAS, RNF43, GNAS, P53*, and *SMAD4* [60, 61].

Algorithmic Approach to Cytological Evaluation of Pancreatic Masses

Indications for pancreatic FNA are the presence of a solid or cystic mass. It is important to distinguish benign, indolent, or inflammatory processes which may be treated with observation, compared to neoplastic processes which require surgery or neoadjuvant or adjuvant chemotherapy. An algorithmic approach in the evaluation of pancreatic lesions includes clinical history, radiographic findings, cytological findings, and ancillary studies to yield the most clinically relevant interpretation of the aspirated material (Fig. 2).

Some of the pancreatic tumors show certain age and gender predilections as MCNs occur in middle-aged women and pancreatoblastoma is a childhood tumor. Imaging findings are very informative as to whether the mass is cystic or solid. This information determines the cytopathological algorithm. Different entities are considered on the radio-graphic information depending on whether the mass is solid, solid and cystic, entirely cystic, or cystic with connection to the pancreatic ductal system. If the lesion is solid, entities such as chronic pancreatitis, lobular atrophy, adenocarcinoma, pancreatic endocrine tumor, ACC, and metastases are some of the main differential diagnoses that are considered. Any solid tumor that undergoes cystic degeneration may present radiographically as a solid and cystic lesion. Tumors that present as solid and cystic lesions include Pan-NETs and SPNs. Purely cystic lesions include MCNs, serous cystadenoma, side branch IPMN, and pseudocysts. When a dilated main pancreatic duct is present or a connection of the cyst to the ductal system is demonstrated, a diagnosis of IPMN may be made. Gross evaluation of the material aspirated is very useful, especially in cystic lesions. Evaluation of the smears starts at a low-power examination where the cellularity, architecture, and background information are collected. At intermediate power, assessments made at low power are confirmed and architectural patterns can be further analyzed. At high power, nuclear and cytological features and mitotic figures are appreciated. Ancillary studies include immunohistochemistry, flow cytometry for suspected lymphoma, cyst fluid analysis for CEA, amylase, and occasionally for *k-RAS* mutations and loss of heterozygosity.

Disclosure Statement

The author has no conflicts of interest to disclose.

References

1 Gill AJ, Klimstra DS, Lam AK, Washington MK: 10 Tumours of the pancreas; in WHO Classification of Tumours Editorial Board: Digestive System Tumours. WHO Classification of Tumours. 5th Edition. Lyon, IARC, 2019, pp 295–372.

2 Rawla P, Sunkara T, Gaduputi V: Epidemiology of pancreatic cancer: global trends, etiology and risk factors. World J Oncol 2019;10:10–27.

3 Bosetti C, Lucenteforte E, Silverman DT, Petersen G, Bracci PM, Ji BT, Negri E, Li D, Risch HA, Olson SH, Gallinger S, Miller AB, Bueno-de-Mesquita HB, Talamini R, Polesel J, Ghadirian P, Baghurst PA, Zatonski W, Fontham E, Bamlet WR, Holly EA, Bertuccio P, Gao YT, Hassan M, Yu H, Kurtz RC, Cotterchio M, Su J, Maisonneuve P, Duell EJ, Boffetta P, La Vecchia C: Cigarette smoking and pancreatic cancer: an analysis from the International Pancreatic Cancer Case-Control Consortium (Panc4). Ann Oncol 2012;23:1880–1888.

4 Michaud DS: Obesity and pancreatic cancer. Recent results. Cancer Res 2016;208:95–105.

5 McWilliams RR, Rabe KG, Olswold C, De Andrade M, Petersen GM: Risk of malignancy in first degree relatives of patients with pancreatic carcinoma. Cancer 2005;104:388–394.

6 Hruban RH, Canto MI, Goggins M, Schulick R, Klein AP: Update on familial pancreatic cancer. Adv Surg 2010;44:293–311.

7 Klein AP, Brune KA, Petersen GM, Goggins M, Tersmette AC, Offerhaus GJ, Griffin C, Cameron JL, Yeo CJ, Kern S, Hruban RH: Prospective risk of pancreatic cancer in familial pancreatic cancer kindreds. Cancer Res 2004;64:2634–2638.

8 Petersen GM: Familial pancreatic cancer. Semin Oncol 2016;43:548–553.

9 Marchegiani G, Crippa S, Malleo G, Partelli S, Capelli P, Pederzoli P, Falconi M: Surgical treatment of pancreatic tumors in childhood and adolescence: uncommon neoplasms with favorable outcome. Pancreatology 2011;11:383–389.

10 La Rosa S, Sessa F, Capella C: Acinar cell carcinoma of the pancreas: overview of clinicopathologic features and insights into the molecular pathology. Front Med 2015;2:41.

11 Barkin J, Vining D, Miale A Jr, Gottlieb S, Redlhammer DE, Kalser MH: Computerized tomography, diagnostic ultrasound, and radionuclide scanning. Comparison of efficacy in diagnosis of pancreatic carcinoma. JAMA 1977;238:2040–2042.

12 Bourbeau D, Sylvestre J, Lévesque HP, Dussault RG, Boivin Y, Dubé S: Computerized axial tomography and fine-needle biopsy in surgery of the pancreas. Can J Surg 1979;22:29–33.

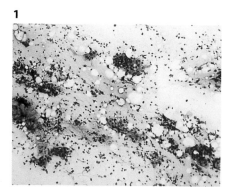
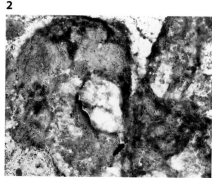

Fig. 1. A well-spread smear – the aspirated material is evenly smeared making it easy to assess the cytological features of the cells. Diff-Quik stain, ×10.

Fig. 2. A thick smear – the aspirated material is entangled in a blood clot making it difficult to assess the cytological features of the cells. Diff-Quik stain, ×10.

spread out on the slide (Fig. 1). Factors causing difficulty in smear interpretation include a bloody smear, a thick smear, and crush artifact (Fig. 2). It is recommended that large clots or tissue fragments be lifted from the smear and submitted for cell block analysis. Thick tissue fragments or clots will not be well visualized on smears.

Rapid On-Site Evaluation

For FNA of solid pancreatic lesions, rapid on-site evaluation (ROSE) has become an integral part of the procedure in many hospitals. Some studies recommend that a cytopathologist/cytotechnologist be present during the procedure for ROSE [2]. There have been several studies suggesting that there is an increase in diagnostic yield and a decreased need for repeat endoscopic ultrasound-guided (EUS)-FNA with ROSE [3–8]. ROSE is said to reduce the probability of false negative and unsatisfactory aspirations. ROSE with EUS-FNA has been reported to provide more accurate diagnoses than EUS-FNA alone [9–11]. ROSE is useful for three different reasons: (i) it helps in the assessment of the adequacy of aspirates to ensure that the lesion is appropriately sampled, (ii) it helps triage the specimen acquired appropriately, based on the initial impression after examining the slides, for additional studies such as flow cytometry, microbiology, or cell block for immunohistochemical stains, and (iii) it provides a provisional diagnosis to the echoendoscopists [11]. Based on this information, a decision is made as to whether additional passes are required or the material collected is sufficient for diagnosis. However, in recent years there have been many studies which have questioned the added benefit of ROSE. Few studies have concluded that the diagnostic yield in unassisted EUS-FNA is not inferior to ROSE-assisted EUS-FNA if at least seven passes are made from the pancreatic lesion [12–15]. A meta-analysis review concluded that ROSE does not improve EUS-FNA adequacy in pancreatic masses [16]. Hence, routine use of ROSE in

EUS-FNA at tertiary cancer centers may not change clinical outcomes. This study also concluded that, since ROSE is a time-consuming service with poor reimbursement and is not available in many centers, it should not be strongly recommended for all EUS-FNA procedures for pancreatic lesions [16]. Non-assisted EUS-FNA procedures incur lower costs and a comparable rate of complications.

Performing ROSE

A staff member from the clinical team/cytotechnologist/cytopathologist assists in specimen collection during the procedure and with smear preparation in the procedure room or suite. At our institution two slides are prepared from each pass. One slide is air dried for Diff-Quik staining and the second slide is fixed in 95% alcohol for later Papanicolaou (PAP) staining in the laboratory. The needle is rinsed in balanced salt solution for cell block processing. The Diff-Quik-stained slide is used for on-site morphological evaluation of adequacy. Additional needle passes are performed based on the assessment of the Diff-Quik-stained smears, and material collected for additional ancillary studies based on the on-site adequacy.

Stains

The stains used for on-site adequacy depend on the institution. Some centers use an alcohol-fixed slide and stain it with rapid hematoxylin and eosin (HE). Other centers may use a rapid PAP or a different type of Romanowsky stain [17]. PAP staining is the standard at most institutions for the alcohol-fixed slides and is used for the final interpretation.

Collection Media

If ancillary studies are needed, additional dedicated passes for cell block material are made. Different types of collection mediums, such as saline, Roswell Park Memorial Institute (RPMI), neutral-buffered formalin, a mixture of formalin

Chapter 2

Published online: September 29, 2020

Centeno BA, Dhillon J (eds): Pancreatic Tumors. Monogr Clin Cytol. Basel, Karger, 2020, vol 26, pp 15–20 (DOI:10.1159/000455730)

Processing of Fine-Needle Aspiration Specimens from Pancreatic Lesions

Jasreman Dhillon[a, b]

Department of Anatomic Pathology, Moffitt Cancer Center, Tampa, FL, USA; Department of Oncologic Sciences and Pathology, University of South Florida, Tampa, FL, USA

Abstract

It is important to adequately process and triage the specimen obtained from fine-needle aspirations (FNAs) of pancreatic lesions. Many echo endoscopists rely on rapid on-site evaluation (ROSE) for adequacy of FNA from solid pancreatic lesions. The role of ROSE in FNA of pancreatic lesions is discussed, as is the triage of material for making smears and cell block preparation. Different techniques of cell block preparation are briefly mentioned. Pancreatic cystic fluid obtained from pancreatic cysts is triaged differently as compared to specimens obtained from solid pancreatic lesions. An algorithmic approach to the processing of pancreatic cystic fluid for molecular and biochemical assays and cytology is discussed. Proper specimen handling is crucial to the accurate interpretation of pancreatic FNA specimens. The methods used to process a sample depend on whether the aspirated sample is solid or cystic and the type of device used for sampling. ROSE has been shown to reduce the number of inadequate specimens and to improve specimen preparation. The details of the various cytological preparation methods available are described in numerous texts. Here we focus on providing a broad overview of specimen collection and processing as it relates to pancreatic FNA, with guidance to the reader based on published and personal experiences.   © 2020 S. Karger AG, Basel

Pancreatic lesions undergoing fine-needle aspiration (FNA) can either be solid or cystic, and this determines the specimen handling. Material aspirated from solid lesions is smeared onto the slides and any extra material aspirated goes for cell block preparation. In contrast, fluid aspirated from cystic lesions is spun down onto the slides and sent for biochemical analysis and molecular testing, details of which are discussed below.

Processing of Cytology Samples from Pancreatic Solid Masses

FNA samples from a solid mass can be prepared by using direct smears, or the sample may be collected directly into a preservative, such as a CytoLyt®, for ThinPrep® processing, or into the SurePath preservative.

Smears

Adequate smear preparation is critical to accurate interpretation. Techniques for adequate smear preparation have been well described in the cytology literature [1]. A good-quality smear shows the cellular material evenly and thinly

46 Pancreatic Section of the British Society of Gastroenterology, Pancreatic Society of Great Britain and Ireland, Association of Upper Gastrointestinal Surgeons of Great Britain and Ireland, Royal College of Pathologists, Special Interest Group for Gastro-Intestinal Radiology: Guidelines for the management of patients with pancreatic cancer periampullary and ampullary carcinomas. Gut 2005;54(suppl V):v1–v16.

47 Tempero MA, Malafa MP, Al-Hawary M, Asbun H, Bain A, Behrman SW, Benson AB, Binder E, Cardin DB, Cha C, Chiorean G, Chung V, Czito B, Dillhoff M, Dotan E, Ferrone CR, Hardacre J, Hawkins WG. National Comprehensive Cancer Network. Pancreatic Adenocarcinoma Version 2.2017. Clinical Practice Guidelines in Oncology. J Natl Compr Canc Netw 2017;15:1028–1061.

48 Sturm PD, Hruban RH, Ramsoekh TB, Noorduyn LA, Tytgat GN, Gouma DJ, Offerhaus GJ: The potential diagnostic use of K-ras codon 12 and p53 alterations in brush cytology from the pancreatic head region. J Pathol 1998;186:247–253.

49 Caldas C, Hahn SA, Hruban RH, Redston MS, Yeo CJ, Kern SE: Detection of K-ras mutations in the stool of patients with pancreatic adenocarcinoma and pancreatic ductal hyperplasia. Cancer Res 1994;54:3568–3573.

50 Tada M, Ohashi M, Shiratori Y, Okudaira T, Komatsu Y, Kawabe T, Yoshida H, Machinami R, Kishi K, Omata M: Analysis of K-ras gene mutation in hyperplastic duct cells of the pancreas without pancreatic disease. Gastroenterology 1996;110:227–231.

51 Yanagisawa A, Ohtake K, Ohashi K, Hori M, Kitagawa T, Sugano H, Kato Y: Frequent c-K-ras oncogene activation in mucous cell hyperplasias of pancreas suffering from chronic inflammation. Cancer Res 1993;53:953–956.

52 Terhune PG, Phifer DM, Tosteson TD, Longnecker DS: K-ras mutation in focal proliferative lesions of human pancreas. Cancer Epidemiol Biomarkers Prev 1998;7:515–521.

53 Hruban RH, Wilentz RE, Kern SE: Genetic progression in the pancreatic ducts. Am J Pathol 2000;156:1821–1825.

54 Levy MJ, Baron TH, Clayton AC, Enders FB, Gostout CJ, Halling KC, Kipp BR, Petersen BT, Roberts LR, Rumalla A, Sebo TJ, Topazian MD, Wiersema MJ, Gores GJ: Prospective evaluation of advanced molecular markers and imaging techniques in patients with indeterminate bile duct strictures. Am J Gastroenterol 2008; 103:1263–1273.

55 Boldorini R, Paganotti A, Sartori M, Allegrini S, Miglio U, Orsello M, Veggiani C, Del Piano M, Monga G: Fluorescence in situ hybridisation in the cytological diagnosis of pancreatobiliary tumours. Pathology 2011;43:335–339.

56 Barr Fritcher EG, Caudill JL, Blue JE, Djuric K, Feipel L, Maritim BK, Ragheb AA, Halling KC, Henry MR, Clayton AC: Identification of malignant cytologic criteria in pancreatobiliary brushings with corresponding positive fluorescence in situ hybridization results. Am J Clin Pathol 2011;136:442–449.

57 Brugge WR, Lewandrowski K, Lee-Lewandrowski E, Centeno BA, Szydlo T, Regan S, del Castillo CF, Warshaw AL: Diagnosis of pancreatic cystic neoplasms: a report of the cooperative pancreatic cyst study. Gastroenterology 2004;126:1330–1336.

58 Wilentz RE, Iacobuzio-Donahue CA, Argani P, McCarthy DM, Parsons JL, Yeo CJ, Kern SE, Hruban RH: Loss of expression of Dpc4 in pancreatic intraepithelial neoplasia: evidence that DPC4 inactivation occurs late in neoplastic progression. Cancer Res 2000;60:2002–2006.

59 Klimstra DS: Pathology reporting of neuroendocrine tumors: essential elements for accurate diagnosis, classification, and staging. Semin Oncol 2013;40:23–36.

60 Wu J, Jiao Y, Dal Molin M, Maitra A, de Wilde RF, Wood LD, Eshleman JR, Goggins MG, Wolfgang CL, Canto MI, Schulick RD, Edil BH, Choti MA, Adsay V, Klimstra DS, Offerhaus GJ, Klein AP, Kopelovich L, Carter H, Karchin R, Allen PJ, Schmidt CM, Naito Y, Diaz LA Jr, Kinzler KW, Papadopoulos N, Hruban RH, Vogelstein B: Whole-exome sequencing of neoplastic cysts of the pancreas reveals recurrent mutations in components of ubiquitin-dependent pathways. Proc Natl Acad Sci USA 2011;108:21188–21193.

61 Kanda M, Knight S, Topazian M, Syngal S, Farrell J, Lee J, Kamel I, Lennon AM, Borges M, Young A, Fujiwara S, Seike J, Eshleman J, Hruban RH, Canto MI, Goggins M: Mutant GNAS detected in duodenal collections of secretin-stimulated pancreatic juice indicates the presence or emergence of pancreatic cysts. Gut 2013;62:1024–1033.

Dr. Jasreman Dhillon
Moffitt Cancer Center
12902 USF Magnolia Drive
Tampa, FL 33612 (USA)
jasreman.dhillon@moffitt.org

13 Legmann P, Vignaux O, Dousset B, Baraza AJ, Palazzo L, Dumontier I, Coste J, Louvel A, Roseau G, Couturier D, Bonnin A: Pancreatic tumors: comparison of dual-phase helical CT and endoscopic sonography. Am J Roentgenol 1998;170: 1315–1322.

14 Graham RA, Bankoff M, Hediger R, Shaker HZ, Reinhold RB: Fine-needle aspiration biopsy of pancreatic ductal adenocarcinoma: loss of diagnostic accuracy with small tumors. J Surg Oncol 1994;55:92–94.

15 Lee JG, Leung JW, Baillie J, Layfield LJ, Cotton PB: Benign, dysplastic, or malignant – making sense of endoscopic bile duct brush cytology: results in 149 consecutive patients. Am J Gastroenterol 1995;90:722–726.

16 Eloubeidi MA, Chen VK, Eltoum IA, Jhala D, Chhieng DC, Jhala N, Vickers SM, Wilcox CM: Endoscopic ultrasound-guided fine needle aspiration biopsy of patients with suspected pancreatic cancer: diagnostic accuracy and acute and 30-day complications. Am J Gastroenterol 2003;98:2663–2668.

17 Wiersema MJ, Vilmann P, Giovannini M, Chang KJ, Wiersema LM: Endosonography-guided fine-needle aspiration biopsy: diagnostic accuracy and complication assessment. Gastroenterology 1997; 112:1087–1095.

18 Williams DB, Sahai AV, Aabakken L, Penman ID, van Velse A, Webb J, Wilson M, Hoffman BJ, Hawes RH: Endoscopic ultrasound guided fine needle aspiration biopsy: a large single center experience. Gut 1999;44:720–726.

19 Yoshinaga S, Suzuki H, Oda I, Saito Y: Role of endoscopic ultrasound-guided fine needle aspiration (EUS-FNA) for diagnosis of solid pancreatic masses. Dig Endosc 2011;23(suppl 1):29–33.

20 Gleeson FC, Kipp BR, Caudill JL, Clain JE, Clayton AC, Halling KC, Henry MR, Rajan E, Topazian MD, Wang KK, Wiersema MJ, Zhang J, Levy MJ: False positive endoscopic ultrasound fine needle aspiration cytology: incidence and risk factors. Gut 2010;59:586–593.

21 Collins BT, Murad FM, Wang JF, Bernadt CT: Rapid on-site evaluation for endoscopic ultrasound-guided fine-needle biopsy of the pancreas decreases the incidence of repeat biopsy procedures. Cancer Cytopathol 2013;121:518–524.

22 Kong F, Zhu J, Kong X, Sun T, Deng X, Du Y, Li Z: Rapid on-site evaluation does not improve endoscopic ultrasound-guided fine needle aspiration adequacy in pancreatic masses: a meta-analysis and systematic review. PLoS One 2016; 11:e0163056.

23 Iglesias-Garcia J, Lariño-Noia J, Abdulkader I, Domínguez-Muñoz JE: Rapid on-site evaluation of endoscopic-ultrasound-guided fine-needle aspiration diagnosis of pancreatic masses. World J Gastroenterol 2014;20:9451–9457.

24 Lee LS, Nieto J, Watson RR, Hwang AL, Muthusamy VR, Walter L, Jajoo K, Ryou MK, Saltzman JR, Saunders MD, Suleiman S, Kadiyala V: Randomized noninferiority trial comparing diagnostic yield of cytopathologist-guided versus 7 passes for endoscopic ultrasound-guided fine-needle aspiration of pancreatic masses. Dig Endosc 2016;28(4): 469–475.

25 Suzuki R, Lee JH, Krishna SG, Ramireddy S, Qiao W, Weston B, Ross WA, Bhutani MS: Repeat endoscopic ultrasound-guided fine needle aspiration for solid pancreatic lesions at a tertiary referral center will alter the initial inconclusive result. J Gastrointest Liver Dis 2013;22:183–187.

26 Gagovic V, Spier B, DeLee R, Barancin C, Lindstrom M, Einstein M, Byrne S, Harter J, Agni R, Pfau PR, Frick TJ, Soni A, Gopal DV: Endoscopic ultrasound fine needle aspiration characteristics of primary adenocarcinoma versus other malignant neoplasms of the pancreas. Can J Gastroenterol 2012;26:691–696.

27 Adler D, Schmidt CM, Al-Haddad M, Barthel JS, Ljung BM, Merchant NB, Romagnuolo J, Shaaban AM, Simeone D, Pitman MB, Layfield LJ: Clinical evaluation, imaging studies, indications for cytologic study and preprocedural requirements for duct brushing studies and pancreatic fine-needle aspiration: The Papanicolaou Society of Cytopathology Guidelines. Cytojournal 2014;11(suppl 1):1.

28 Pitman MB, Centeno BA, Ali SZ, Genevay M, Stelow E, Mino-Kenudson M, Castillo CF, Schmidt CM, Brugge WR, Layfield LJ: Standardized terminology and nomenclature for pancreatobiliary cytology: The Papanicolaou Society of Cytopathology Guidelines. Diagn Cytopathol 2014;42:338–350.

29 Layfield LJ, Ehya H, Filie AC, Hruban RH, Jhala N, Joseph L, Vielh P, Pitman MB: Utilization of ancillary studies in the cytologic diagnosis of biliary and pancreatic lesions: The Papanicolaou Society of Cytopathology Guidelines. Cytojournal 2014; 11(suppl 1):4.

30 Kurtycz DF, Field A, Tabatabai L, Michaels C, Young N, Schmidt CM, Farrell J, Gopal D, Simeone D, Merchant NB, Pitman MB: Post-brushing and fine-needle aspiration biopsy follow-up and treatment options for patients with pancreatobiliary lesions: The Papanicolaou Society of Cytopathology Guidelines. Cytojournal 2014;11(suppl 1): 5.

31 Brugge WR, De Witt J, Klapman JB, Ashfaq R, Shidham V, Chhieng D, Kwon R, Baloch Z, Zarka M, Staerkel G: Techniques for cytologic sampling of pancreatic and bile duct lesions: The Papanicolaou Society of Cytopathology Guidelines. Cytojournal 2014;11(suppl 1):2.

32 Tanaka M, Fernández-del Castillo C, Adsay V, Chari S, Falconi M, Jang JY, Kimura W, Levy P, Pitman MB, Schmidt CM, Shimizu M, Wolfgang CL, Yamaguchi K, Yamao K: International consensus guidelines 2012 for the management of IPMN and MCN of the pancreas. Pancreatology 2012;12:183–197.

33 Tanaka M, Fernández-Del Castillo C, Kamisawa T, Jang JY, Levy P, Ohtsuka T, Salvia R, Shimizu Y, Tada M, Wolfgang CL: Revisions of international consensus Fukuoka guidelines for the management of IPMN of the pancreas. Pancreatology 2017;17:738–753.

34 Howard TJ, Chin AC, Streib EW, Kopecky KK, Wiebke EA: Value of helical computed tomography, angiography, and endoscopic ultrasound in determining resectability of periampullary carcinoma. Am J Surg 1997;174:237–241.

35 Midwinter MJ, Beveridge CJ, Wilsdon JB, Bennett MK, Baudouin CJ, Charnley RM: Correlation between spiral computed tomography, endoscopic ultrasonography and findings at operation in pancreatic and ampullary tumours. Br J Surg 1999;86: 189–193.

36 Mertz HR, Sechopoulos P, Delbeke D, Leach SD: EUS, PET, and CT scanning for evaluation of pancreatic adenocarcinoma. Gastrointest Endosc 2000;52:367–371.

37 Vilmann P, Săftoiu A: Endoscopic ultrasound-guided fine needle aspiration biopsy: equipment and technique. J Gastroenterol Hepatol 2006;21: 1646–1655.

38 Lee JH, Stewart J, Ross WA, Anandasabapathy S, Xiao L, Staerkel G: Blinded prospective comparison of the performance of 22-gauge and 25-gauge needles in endoscopic ultrasound-guided fine needle aspiration of the pancreas and peri-pancreatic lesions. Dig Dis Sci 2009;54:2274–2281.

39 Kubiliun N, Ribeiro A, Fan YS, Rocha-Lima CM, Sleeman D, Merchan J, Barkin J, Levi J: EUS-FNA with rescue fluorescence in situ hybridization for the diagnosis of pancreatic carcinoma in patients with inconclusive on-site cytopathology results. Gastrointest Endosc 2011;74:541–547.

40 Amato E, Molin MD, Mafficini A, Yu J, Malleo G, Rusev B, Fassan M, Antonello D, Sadakari Y, Castelli P, Zamboni G, Maitra A, Salvia R, Hruban RH, Bassi C, Capelli P, Lawlor RT, Goggins M, Scarpa A: Targeted next-generation sequencing of cancer genes dissects the molecular profiles of intraductal papillary neoplasms of the pancreas. J Pathol 2014;233:217–227.

41 Layfield LJ, Schmidt RL, Hirschowitz SL, Olson MT, Ali SZ, Dodd LL: Significance of the diagnostic categories "atypical" and "suspicious for malignancy" in the cytologic diagnosis of solid pancreatic masses. Diagn Cytopathol 2014;42:292–296.

42 Layfield LJ, Dodd L, Factor R, Schmidt RL: Malignancy risk associated with diagnostic categories defined by the Papanicolaou Society of Cytopathology pancreaticobiliary guidelines. Cancer Cytopathol 2014;122:420–427.

43 Abdelgawwad MS, Alston E, Eltoum IA: The frequency and cancer risk associated with the atypical cytologic diagnostic category in endoscopic ultrasound-guided fine-needle aspiration specimens of solid pancreatic lesions: a meta-analysis and argument for a Bethesda system for reporting cytopathology of the pancreas. Cancer Cytopathol 2013;121:620–628.

44 Roland CL, Bian A, Mansour JC, Yopp AC, Balch GC, Sharma A, Xie XJ, Schwarz RE: Survival impact of malignant pancreatic neuroendocrine and islet cell neoplasm phenotypes. J Surg Oncol 2012; 105:595–600.

45 Yamaguchi K, Tanaka M; Committee for Revision of Clinical Guidelines for Pancreatic Cancer of Japan Pancreas Society: EBM based clinical guidelines for pancreatic cancer 2009 from the Japan Pancreas Society: a synopsis. Jpn J Clin Oncol 2011;41:836–840.

and 95% ethanol, and methanol, are available and can be utilized for needle rinses. Specimens collected in saline and RPMI can be used for flow cytometry if needed. Needle rinses can be processed into cell blocks or cytospin slides if the material collected is scant. Needle rinses collected in preservatives containing alcohol (methanol in PreservCyt and ethanol in SurePath Preservative Fluid) can be processed using ThinPrep® and SurePath™ respectively. Although ThinPrep preparation is being used for pancreatic FNAs, there are certain pitfalls and limitations to it. It is difficult to recognize mucin on ThinPrep slides and mucinous neoplasms may be incorrectly diagnosed. A study by de Luna et al. [18] concluded that the diagnostic accuracy of pancreatic FNA using ThinPrep is inferior to that of conventional smears. However, ThinPrep® remains a viable substitute for smear preparation for practices in which a cytologist is not available on-site to prepare the slides. At our institution, we receive pancreatic FNA specimens submitted directly into CytoLyt, and have found them to have a good diagnostic yield. Aspirates form cysts have been identified to have background mucin and the epithelium is well preserved.

Cell Blocks
A good cell block preparation can be utilized for additional ancillary studies such as immunohistochemical stains, fluorescence in situ hybridization, and other molecular studies necessary for the diagnosis and treatment of the patients. Ancillary tests that are validated for formalin-fixed specimens may have to be revalidated for specimens that are fixed in alcohol. Alcohol-fixed specimens may have altered antigenicity which may render some of the tests falsely negative.

Different cell block preparation methods utilize different collection mediums for transportation and fixation of the specimen collected, for example methanol is used as a fixative for the automated Cellient cell block technique [19]. Other methods of cell block preparation are the clot and scrape method, BBC cell block fixative method, plasma thrombin cell block preparation, collodion bag cell block procedure, Shandon cytoblock method, HistoGel method, Tissue coagulum clot method, and Formalin or alcohol vapor method [19]. The clot and scrape method and formalin/alcohol vapor method are both inexpensive techniques but are reported to have variable quality and cellularity. The collodion method, although time consuming, has a good cellular yield, making it ideal for samples with scant cellularity. Collodion is admixed with an ether-based solvent; it must be handled in a laminar flow hood and stored in small volumes in a flameproof enclosure [20]. The Cellient automated system is time consuming and expensive but is great for small/scanty samples and provides a crisp cellular architecture. As it is fully automated, there is little chance of cross-contamination. It utilizes methanol as the fixative which could interfere with certain immunohistochemical stains. However, in a separate protocol formalin can be used as the fixative. The instrument can accommodate only one specimen block at a time, so high-volume labs may require multiple instruments. The HistoGel method is tedious but helps in the concentration of cells and provides good cellular preservation. The plasma thrombin method is an inexpensive and simple method and provides a clean background. The disadvantages of this technique include an inability to control clot formation and irregular distribution of cells within the pellet. Some thromboplastin agents contain epithelial cells that may interfere with the diagnosis and with the interpretation of ancillary studies [21].

Processing of Cytology Samples from Pancreatic Cystic Lesions

The goal of pancreatic cyst fluid evaluation is to differentiate mucin from non-mucinous lesions, and to identify cysts carrying a high-risk malignancy [22, 23]. Hence, both symptomatic and asymptomatic pancreatic cysts are actively evaluated to determine the nature of the cyst. It is extremely crucial to examine the cyst fluid aspirated to make this distinction and to rule out high-grade dysplasia or adenocarcinoma associated with the cyst.

Pancreatic cyst fluids need to be submitted fresh and undiluted. The pancreatic cyst fluid needs to be triaged for biochemical analysis, to include carcinoembryonic antigen (CEA) and amylase, and for molecular analysis, in addition to cytology. CEA and amylase can be performed from the supernatant, which is preferred, as it preserves the cells in the specimen for cytological evaluation.

Chai et al. [24] developed a volume-based protocol using minimal pancreatic cyst fluid volumes for biochemical, molecular, and cytology analysis. The addition of molecular analysis to the traditional CEA and cytological examination of the pancreatic cyst fluid has led to a reappraisal of how these samples are triaged and the comparative roles of these different modalities [25, 26]. Ideally, if the cyst fluid volume is sufficient it is split into neat (unaltered fluid), smears, cell block, and supernatant fluid. Chai et al. [24] proposed the following pancreatic cyst fluid triage based on volume:

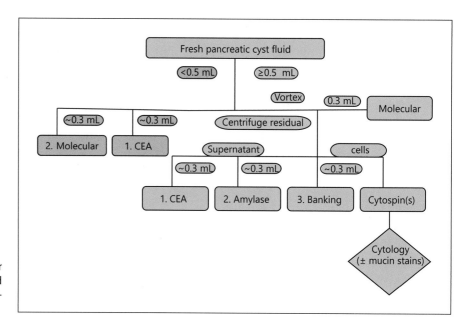

Fig. 3. A volume-dependent protocol for processing of aspirated pancreatic cyst fluid [28] (reproduced with permission from Cambridge University Press).

1. Volume ≤1 mL
   (a) Centrifuge the specimen for generating supernatant fluid and deposit (pellet)
   (b) Deposit to process as a cell block for cytology review and *KRAS* testing
   (c) Supernatant fluid (0.5 mL) to biochemistry for CEA
   (d) Remaining supernatant fluid frozen and stored
2. Volume >1 mL
   (a) Neat fluid (0.5 mL) to biochemistry for CEA
   (b) Centrifuge specimen to generate deposit and supernatant fluid
   (c) Deposit to process as a cell block and 2 wet-fixed smears
   (d) Supernatant and any excess neat fluid frozen and stored
   (e) *KRAS* mutation testing on cell block material
   (f) For difficult cases *KRAS* retesting can be performed on stored supernatant and/or neat fluid

A limitation of this proposal is that it only includes CEA measurements, and uses neat fluid for CEA measurements if the volume is greater than 1 mL. Also, *KRAS* is the only mutation evaluated. Current analyses include a greater number of targets.

A protocol proposed by Dr. Pitman calls for only using the supernatant for CEA and amylase, and preserving the neat fluid for cytology and molecular testing (Fig. 3). This protocol is also volume dependent.

1. Volume <0.5 mL
   (a) Divide in equal halves for molecular testing and CEA level
2. Volume ≥0.5 mL
   (a) Vortex the specimen and remove 0.3 mL for molecular assessment
   (b) Centrifuge the remaining fluid; send the supernatant for CEA and amylase levels, and the remainder for cytology

The ideal protocol for cyst fluid processing may be laboratory dependent. The CEA and amylase may be processed from the supernatant. Therefore, it is not necessary to send the neat fluid. Recent studies have shown DNA retrieval from residual cytological material, so it may be possible to perform a limited mutational panel on the cyst fluid supernatant.

Cytology is the most sensitive test for determining malignancy in pancreatic cysts [27]. However, cytology is hampered by low cellularity and the presence of degenerative changes. The presence or absence of background mucin and high-grade dysplasia should be reported. Finally, it is a combination of CT/MRI findings, molecular test results, CEA and amylase levels, and cytological features present on slides and/or cell block sections that determine the final diagnosis rendered and subsequent surgical/non-surgical management of the patients.

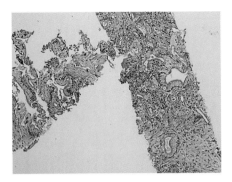

Fig. 4. Biopsy cores obtained from a pancreatic solid mass showing infiltrating glands. HE stain, ×10.

Next-Generation Biopsy Devices

Factors influencing the diagnostic yield of a lesion include the location, size, nature of the lesion (solid, cystic, or firm), and the type and the size of the needle used for aspiration. Needle types with different tip designs that have been intro-

duced for solid masses include the EchoTip ProCore® HD Ultrasound (Cook Medical, Bloomington, IN), Shark core™ FNB Exchange (Medtronic, Minneapolis, MN), and the Acquire™ (Boston Scientific, Marlborough, MA). These newer-generation EUS-FNA biopsy needles help obtain small histopathology specimens from pancreatic solid masses (Fig. 4). For pancreatic cystic masses the Moray micro forceps have been used. These needles not only improve the tissue yield compared to FNA, but also significantly reduce the number of passes and provide a larger amount of cellularity for diagnostic accuracy and ancillary studies. In our experience, material obtained from these newer-generation needles, depending on the gauge of the needle used and the experience of the laboratory, is best processed using cell blocks as the biopsies are fragile and fragment easily.

Disclosure Statement

The author has no conflicts of interest to disclose.

References

1 Al-Abbadi MA: Basics of cytology. Avicenna J Med 2011;1:18–28.
2 Klapman JB, Logrono R, Dye CE, Waxman I: Clinical impact of on-site cytopathology interpretation on endoscopic ultrasoundguided fine needle aspiration. Am J Gastroenterol 2003;98:1289–1294.
3 Hebert-Magee S, Bae S, Varadarajulu S, et al: The presence of a cytopathologist increases the diagnostic accuracy of endoscopic ultrasound-guided fine needle aspiration cytology for pancreatic adenocarcinoma: a meta-analysis. Cytopathology 2013;24:159–171.
4 Schmidt RL, Walker BS, Howard K, Layfield LJ, Adler DG: Rapid on-site evaluation increases endoscopic ultrasound-guided fine-needle aspiration adequacy for pancreatic lesions. Dig Dis Sci 2013;58:872–882.
5 Haba S, Yamao K, Bhatia V, et al: Diagnostic ability and factors affecting accuracy of endoscopic ultrasound-guided fine needle aspiration for pancreatic solid lesions: Japanese large single center experience. J Gastroenterol 2013;48:973–981.
6 Collins BT, Murad FM, Wang JF, Bernadt CT: Rapid on-site evaluation for endoscopic ultrasound-guided fine-needle biopsy of the pancreas decreases the incidence of repeat biopsy procedures. Cancer Cytopathol 2013;121:518–524.
7 Iglesias-Garcia J, Dominguez-Munoz JE, Abdulkader I, et al: Influence of on-site cytopathology evaluation on the diagnostic accuracy of endoscopic ultrasound-guided fine needle aspiration (EUS-FNA) of solid pancreatic masses. Am J Gastroenterol 2011;106:1705–1710.

8 Ecka RS, Sharma M: Rapid on-site evaluation of EUS-FNA by cytopathologist: an experience of a tertiary hospital. Diagn Cytopathol 2013;41:1075–1080.
9 Chang KJ: Maximizing the yield of EUS-guided fine-needle aspiration. Gastrointest Endosc 2002; 56:S28–S34.
10 Yamao K, Sawaki A, Mizuno N, Shimizu Y, Yatabe Y, Koshikawa T: Endoscopic ultrasound-guided fine-needle aspiration biopsy (EUS-FNAB): past, present, and future. J Gastroenterol 2005;40: 1013–1023.
11 Logrono R, Waxman I: Interactive role of the cytopathologists in EUS-guided fine needle aspiration: an effective approach. Gastrointest Endosc 2001;54:485–490.
12 Erickson RA, Sayage-Rabie L, Beissner RS: Factors predicting the number of EUS-guided fine-needle passes for diagnosis of pancreatic malignancies. Gastrointest Endosc 2000;51:184–190.
13 LeBlanc JK, Ciaccia D, Al-Assi MT, et al: Optimal number of EUS-guided fine needle passes needed to obtain a correct diagnosis. Gastrointest Endosc 2004;59:475–481.
14 Storch I, Jorda M, Thurer R, et al: Advantage of EUS Trucut biopsy combined with fine-needle aspiration without immediate on-site cytopathologic examination. Gastrointest Endosc 2006;64: 505–511.

15 Lee LS, Nieto J, Watson RR, Hwang AL, Muthusamy VR, Walter L, Jajoo K, Ryou MK, Saltzman JR, Saunders MD, Suleiman S, Kadiyala V: Randomized noninferiority trial comparing diagnostic yield of cytopathologist-guided versus 7 passes for EUS-FNA of pancreatic masses. Dig Endosc 2016; 28:469–475.
16 Kong F, Zhu J, Kong X, Sun T, Deng X, Du Y, Li Z: Rapid on-site evaluation does not improve endoscopic ultrasound-guided fine needle aspiration adequacy in pancreatic masses: a meta-analysis and systematic review. PLoS One 2016; 11:e0163056.
17 Thakur M, Guttikonda VR: Modified ultrafast Papanicolaou staining technique: a comparative study. J Cytol 2017;34:149–153.
18 de Luna R, Eloubeidi MA, Sheffield MV, Eltoum I, Jhala N, Jhala D, Chen VK, Chhieng DC: Comparison of ThinPrep and conventional preparations in pancreatic fine-needle aspiration biopsy. Diagn Cytopathol 2004;30:71–76.
19 Rollins SD, Russell DK: Cytopathology in focus: cell blocks: getting the most from the least invasive method. CAP Today, Aug 2017.
20 Balassanian R, Wool GD, Ono JC, Olejnik-Nave J, Mah MM, Sweeney BJ, Liberman H, Ljung BM, Pitman MB: A superior method for cell block preparation for fine-needle aspiration biopsies. Cancer Cytopathol 2016;124:508–518.
21 Henwood AF, Charlton A: Extraneous epithelial cells from thromboplastin in cell blocks. Cytopathology 2014;25:412–413.

22 Pitman MB, Lewandrowski K, Shen J, Sahani D, Brugge W, Fernandez-del Castillo C. Pancreatic cysts: preoperative diagnosis and clinical management. Cancer Cytopathol. 2010;118(1):1–13.

23 Tanaka M, Chari S, Adsay V, Fernandez-del Castillo C, Falconi M, Shimizu M, Yamaguchi K, Yamao K, Matsuno S; International Association of Pancreatology: International consensus guidelines for management of intraductal papillary mucinous neoplasms and mucinous cystic neoplasms of the pancreas. Pancreatology 2006;6:17–32.

24 Chai SM, Herba K, Kumarasinghe MP, de Boer WB, Amanuel B, Grieu-Iacopetta F, Lim EM, Segarajasingam D, Yusoff I, Choo C, Frost F: Optimizing the multimodal approach to pancreatic cyst fluid diagnosis: developing a volume-based triage protocol. Cancer Cytopathol 2013;121:86–100.

25 Khalid A, McGrath KM, Zahid M, Wilson M, Brody D, Swalsky P, Moser AJ, Lee KK, Slivka A, Whitcomb DC, Finkelstein S: The role of pancreatic cyst fluid molecular analysis in predicting cyst pathology. Clin Gastroenterol Hepatol 2005;3:967–973.6.

26 Khalid A, Zahid M, Finkelstein SD, LeBlanc JK, Kaushik N, Ahmad N, Brugge WR, Edmundowicz SA, Hawes RH, McGrath KM: Pancreatic cyst fluid DNA analysis in evaluating pancreatic cysts: a report of the PANDA study. Gastrointest Endosc 2009;69:1095–1102.

27 Cizginer S, Turner B, Bilge AR, Karaca C, Pitman MB, Brugge WR: Cyst fluid carcinoembryonic antigen is an accurate diagnostic marker of pancreatic mucinous cysts. Pancreas 2011;40:1024–1028.

28 Centeno BA, Stelow EB, Pitman MB (eds): Pancreatic Cytohistology. Cambridge, Cambridge University Press, 2015, chapt 3, p 30.

Dr. Jasreman Dhillon
Moffitt Cancer Center
12902 USF Magnolia Drive
Tampa, FL 33612 (USA)
jasreman.dhillon@moffitt.org

Chapter 3

Published online: September 29, 2020

Centeno BA, Dhillon J (eds): Pancreatic Tumors. Monogr Clin Cytol. Basel, Karger, 2020, vol 26, pp 21–33 (DOI:10.1159/000455731)

Imaging of Pancreatic Tumors

Brian Morse[a, b]   Jason Klapman[b, c]

[a]Department of Diagnostic Imaging, Moffitt Cancer Center, Tampa, FL, USA; [b]Department of Oncologic Science, University of South Florida, Tampa, FL, USA; [c]Department of Gastrointestinal Oncology, Moffitt Cancer Center, Tampa, FL, USA

Abstract

Imaging plays a key role in the diagnosis and staging of pancreatic tumors. Imaging modalities utilized for the evaluation of pancreatic tumors include: transabdominal and endoscopic ultrasound, computed tomography, and magnetic resonance imaging. Each of these modalities has different strengths and weaknesses which must be considered in the setting of evaluating a pancreatic tumor. Imaging can determine if a pancreatic tumor is cystic or solid and help develop a differential diagnosis based on the lesion's imaging features. If a malignant pancreatic tumor is diagnosed, imaging can assist with initial staging by determining the size and local extent of the tumor as well as evaluating for nodal and metastatic disease. Here we review the different imaging modalities utilized to evaluate pancreatic masses, describe the key imaging features of the most significant entities in the differential diagnosis, and describe the diagnostic imaging approach.
© 2020 S. Karger AG, Basel

Imaging Techniques

Imaging of the pancreas can be performed with transabdominal ultrasound (TUS), computed tomography (CT), endoscopic ultrasound (EUS), or magnetic resonance imaging (MRI). There are advantages and disadvantages to all of these imaging modalities (Table 1).

TUS is a quick and low-cost way to evaluate the pancreas. However, because the transducer is external to the patient, the ultrasound energy is attenuated by overlying soft tissues which results in a degraded image quality. This has become more of an issue with TUS over the past decades as obesity continues to increase in incidence. Gas in the bowel can essentially block the ultrasound energy which may render the exam non-diagnostic. This is particularly a concern when evaluating the pancreas, which is deeper in the abdomen than other structures. Air in the adjacent stomach and duodenum can significantly degrade the pancreatic evaluation by TUS. Ultrasound can distinguish a solid lesion from a cystic lesion, but this may be hampered by an abundance of overlying soft tissues. TUS also offers little information about tumor stage compared to other modalities. As CT and MRI technology has continued to improve, TUS plays more of a role in lesion detection rather than characterization.

CT is widely available and provides a fast, comprehensive evaluation of pancreatic lesions. When CT is performed to evaluate the pancreas a dedicated "pancreas protocol" CT should be employed. The exact details of the exam will vary at individual sites, but the exam should include multiphase imaging and high spatial resolution mul-

Table 1. Comparison of imaging modalities used to evaluate pancreatic masses

Modality	Advantages	Disadvantages
TUS	Quick, widely available Relatively inexpensive	Often cannot visualize entire pancreas May have difficulty with lesion characterization
CT	Quick, widely available Can classify as cystic or solid (IV contrast may be required) Excellent spatial resolution (staging cancer, MPD communication, etc.)	Ionizing radiation Contrast use limited with poor renal function
MRI	Easily distinguishes cystic from solid lesions Probably the best for evaluation of cystic lesions No ionizing radiation, contrast material not nephrotoxic	Longer exam time, expensive Susceptible to artifacts Contrast use prohibited with very poor renal function
EUS	Highly sensitive and specific for pancreas diseases Has the ability to perform FNA or biopsy at the same time	Invasive test requiring sedation Expensive Operator dependent

tiplanar imaging. Multiphase imaging refers to the acquisition of multiple scans of the abdomen at different times, typically before contrast administration and then in the pancreatic phase and portal venous phase. Pancreatic phase imaging results in the highest level of pancreatic enhancement and also allows a good evaluation of the arteries of the pancreas [1, 2]. Images should be acquired at the highest spatial resolution possible to allow reformatting into coronal and sagittal planes in addition to standard axial images. This optimized protocol will allow detection and characterization of pancreatic tumors and staging in cases of pancreatic malignancy. CT does employ ionizing radiation, so it should be used only when appropriate, and MRI would be preferred when radiation exposure is suboptimal (e.g., younger patients, imaging during pregnancy). The iodinated contrast used with CT can also cause idiosyncratic reactions and should be used cautiously with impaired renal function.

MRI is not as widely available as CT but also excels in the evaluation of pancreatic tumors. MRI is more sensitive than CT for the evaluation of subtle enhancement and can provide a more detailed picture of the biliary and pancreatic ductal anatomy [3]. The disadvantages of MRI include cost, exam time, and susceptibility to artifacts. When MRI is used to evaluate the pancreas, magnetic resonance cholangiopancreatography (MRCP) may be employed. MRCP imaging utilizes heavily T2-weighted images to produce detailed images of the biliary system and main pancreatic duct, typi-

cally in multiple imaging planes, resulting in a more sensitive evaluation of pathology [4].

EUS is an imaging modality that was originally developed in the 1980s in part to overcome the limitations of TUS evaluation of the pancreas where the overlying bowel gas pattern would obscure viewing the pancreas routinely. EUS is an endoscopic procedure that uses ultrasound waves to view the pancreas through the stomach and duodenum. It is an extremely sensitive and specific test for evaluating the pancreas, especially for detecting lesions of less than 2 cm, which may be missed on CT scan or MRI. Another advantage that EUS has over other imaging modalities is the ability to perform fine-needle aspiration (FNA) or needle biopsy at the same time as the imaging assessment. As a result, EUS has become integral in the work-up and diagnosis of pancreatic solid and cystic masses. The main disadvantage to performing EUS is that it is an invasive procedure that requires sedation and has rare adverse events associated with it, especially in instances where FNA or fine-needle biopsy is performed. An example of the utility of EUS in evaluating a patient with a dilated pancreatic duct without a visible mass on CT scan is shown in Figure 1.

PET/CT using fluorodeoxyglucose (FDG) has limited utility in the diagnosis of pancreatic lesions. FDG PET/CT can be used with pancreatic ductal carcinoma in staging and assessing the response to therapy, but has little utility in detecting or classifying pancreatic lesions overall. Some utility has been reported with PET/CT in distinguishing benign

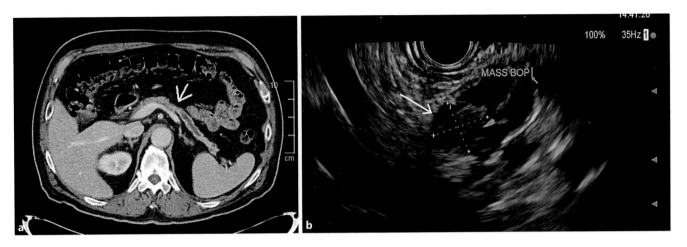

Fig. 1. Pancreatic mass seen by EUS, but not detected by CT scan. **a** CT scan showing a dilated duct but no obvious mass (arrow). **b** EUS imaging shows a 12-mm mass (arrow) causing the pancreatic duct dilation. FNA was performed and positive for adenocarcinoma.

Table 2. Imaging differential diagnosis of hypervascular pancreatic masses identified on CT scan

Neuroendocrine tumor	Functional tumors will have relevant clinical signs/symptoms
	May employ functional imaging (OctreoScan ^{68}Ga-DOTA agents)
Metastases	History of cancer, particularly renal cell carcinoma
Serous cystadenoma	Not solid but, when small, numerous enhancing septations can mimic solid mass
Intrapancreatic splenule	Mimics the appearance of spleen by CT or MRI
	Can verify splenic tissue with nuclear medicine imaging

from malignant pancreatic cysts, but this can be accomplished with less expensive imaging methods [5].

Approach to Imaging Evaluation

The first step in the imaging analysis of pancreatic tumors is determining if the lesion is solid or cystic. At TUS a cystic lesion will appear black or grayish (anechoic or hypoechoic) relative to adjacent normal pancreatic parenchyma, depending on the internal complexity of the lesion. If Doppler imaging is employed there should be no central blood flow (there may be a small amount of flow within internal septations). Of course, this assumes there is no bowel gas blocking the ultrasound beam, a frequent occurrence in the pancreatic head and body. It may also be difficult to distinguish a microcystic lesion from a solid lesion by TUS. At CT cystic and solid lesions are distinguished by their density and postcontrast enhancement. The density of a cystic lesion will be similar to fluid (0–20 HU) whereas a solid lesion will have a higher density. After the administration of IV contrast a solid lesion will increase in density (i.e., enhancement) whereas a cystic lesion does not change (although cystic lesions with complex internal architecture can enhance). Clear evidence of enhancement allows the definitive diagnosis of a solid lesion. Cystic lesions have a very high signal on T2-weighted MRI images. Solid lesions have a lower signal on T2-weighted images and enhance after contrast administration. Identifying a lesion as solid or cystic at imaging is the first step in developing a differential diagnosis and looking for features that might suggest a specific diagnosis or identify a malignant lesion.

Solid Lesions

Once it is determined that a pancreatic lesion is solid, the differential can be refined based on other imaging features. A good starting point is the enhancement pattern at multiphase imaging. "Hypervascular" lesions are lesions which enhance more than normal pancreas on early postcontrast images (Table 2). Hypervascular lesions include: pancreatic neuroendocrine tumors (PanNETs; Fig. 2), metastases (particularly renal cell carcinoma), serous cystadenoma, and intrapancreatic splenule [6]. Serous cystadenoma is a cystic lesion, but the internal septations enhance, and therefore if the

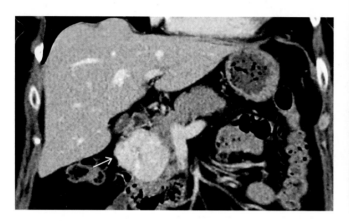

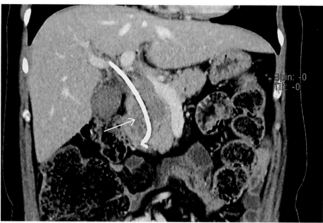

Fig. 2. Hypervascular mass. Coronal CT image shows a hypervascular mass in the head of the pancreas (indicated by the arrow). This mass was a pancreatic neuroendocrine tumor but other lesions in the differential for a hypervascular pancreatic mass could have a similar appearance.

Fig. 3. Primary pancreatic lymphoma. The arrow indicates a hypovascular mass in the head of the pancreas. There is a plastic common bile duct stent in place. Biopsy revealed primary lymphoma of the pancreas, but pancreatic ductal adenocarcinoma could have an identical appearance.

Table 3. Imaging differential diagnosis of hypovascular pancreatic masses identified on CT scan

Ductal adenocarcinoma	Obstructs main pancreatic duct
	Frequently involves adjacent vasculature
	Relevant symptoms, tumor markers
Metastases	History of cancer
Ampullary carcinoma	Can mimic pancreatic mass
Neuroendocrine tumor	Nonfunctional tumors may grow to become large and heterogeneous at time of detection
Lymphoma	Look for other signs of lymphoma, e.g., widespread lymphadenopathy
Solid pseudopapillary neoplasm	Encapsulated, internal blood products

lesion is very small is can look like a solid lesion at TUS or CT. It will also look solid on postcontrast MRI images, but MRI should offer other clues to the cystic morphology. Metastases enter the differential if the patient has a history of cancer. Renal cell cancer is one of the most common tumors to metastasize to the pancreas and these metastases almost always appear hypervascular. PanNETs are hypervascular, with the exception that non-functional tumors may grow to be large before detection and these could show more heterogeneous enhancement or central cystic/necrotic change. If the lesion is in the tail of the pancreas an intrapancreatic splenule should be considered. These lesions parallel the appearance of the adjacent spleen on multiphase CT and also mirror the spleen signal on all MRI sequences. Nuclear medicine imaging with sulfur colloid scintigraphy or tagged red blood cells may help clinch this diagnosis in equivocal cases.

"Hypovascular" pancreatic tumors enhance less than normal pancreatic parenchyma on multiphase imaging (Table 3). These tumors include: ductal adenocarcinoma (PDAC), metastases, ampullary carcinoma (in the head of the pancreas), PanNETs (less common, large, typically nonfunctional), lymphoma (uncommon), solid pseudopapillary neoplasm (SPN), among other lesions [6, 7]. The differential for a hypovascular pancreatic mass is more extensive and there are fewer clinical and imaging clues which can clinch a diagnosis without tissue sampling. PDAC typically manifests as a focal, hypoenhancing mass which obstructs the main pancreatic duct. PDAC may be difficult to visualize by CT or MRI and the lesions can be very poorly defined. A meticulous technique including multiphase imaging with pancreatic phase and thin-section, multiplanar reconstructions are necessary for adequate detection and tumor delin-

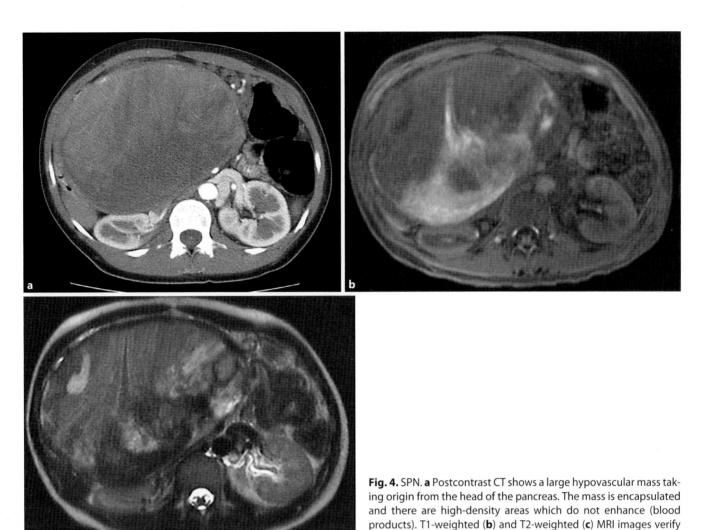

Fig. 4. SPN. **a** Postcontrast CT shows a large hypovascular mass taking origin from the head of the pancreas. The mass is encapsulated and there are high-density areas which do not enhance (blood products). T1-weighted (**b**) and T2-weighted (**c**) MRI images verify the capsule and internal blood products. The patient was a young female; all features were compatible with SPN.

eation. There are also clinical features which can suggest the diagnosis along with the typical imaging features (strong family history, abdominal pain and weight loss, elevated CA19-9). Metastases to the pancreas are less common than PDAC but are also generally hypovascular. A history of malignancy raises this possibility, with melanoma, lung, and breast cancer some of the most common tumors to metastasize to the pancreas [6]. If the mass is located in the head of the pancreas it may be difficult to distinguish PDAC from ampullary cancer. Lymphoma can involve the pancreas as primary pancreatic lymphoma or tumor which spreads from another location to involve the pancreas [8]. Primary lymphoma of the pancreas is much less common and the two can usually be distinguished based on the clinical history and other imaging findings [9]. For example, if there is

tumor involving the pancreas with widespread lymphadenopathy then it is not primary pancreatic lymphoma. Otherwise, primary pancreatic lymphoma can closely mimic PDAC [10] (Fig. 3). SPN is typically an encapsulated mass with internal blood products but can exhibit atypical features which many times preclude a diagnosis without tissue sampling [11] (Fig. 4). Just based on this brief discussion it is evident that hypovascular masses are much more difficult to definitively characterize by imaging alone. A further complication is that rare pancreatic tumors, such as acinar cell carcinoma, also typically appear hypovascular [6]. When evaluating a hypovascular pancreatic tumor, clinical features (age, sex, symptoms) and tumor markers play an important role in narrowing the differential. In most cases tissue sampling is necessary to make a diagnosis.

Table 4. NCCN resectability criteria for PDAC based on imaging studies

Resectable	No tumor contact with the celiac axis, common hepatic artery, or superior mesenteric artery
	No tumor contact with the portal vein or superior mesenteric vein
Borderline resectable	Tumor contacts the common hepatic artery but can be resected with artery reconstruction
	Tumor contacts the superior mesenteric artery but involves ≤180 degrees of the circumference
	Tumor contacts the celiac axis but involves ≤180 degrees of the circumference
	Tumor contacts the portal vein or superior mesenteric vein but can be resected with vein reconstruction
	Tumor contacts the inferior vena cava
Unresectable	Distant metastatic disease is present
	Tumor contact with the celiac axis or superior mesenteric artery >180 degrees
	Tumor involvement of portal vein or superior mesenteric vein which is unreconstructible after tumor resection

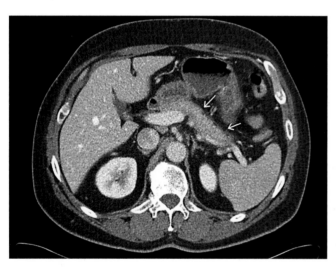

Fig. 5. Autoimmune pancreatitis. The pancreas shows loss of the normal lobulated architecture and a rim of hypoenhancing tissue (indicated by arrows) in this case of AIP.

There are also important mimics of pancreatic tumor which must be considered in the work-up of a hypovascular pancreatic mass. These include autoimmune pancreatitis (AIP), pseudo-mass of acute/chronic pancreatitis, groove pancreatitis, and focal fatty infiltration [6]. Typical features of AIP affecting the pancreas are loss of normal pancreatic architecture, a hypoenhancing rim around the pancreas, and non-specific lesions in other organs [12] (Fig. 5). There are two types of AIP and both types commonly involve the pancreas. Type 1 AIP is the pancreatic manifestation of a systemic process, IgG4-related disease [12]. Serum IgG4

levels are commonly elevated with type 1 AIP. Type 2 only affects the pancreas and is more common in younger patients [12]. Caution must be utilized when evaluating cases of acute or chronic pancreatitis because inflammatory deformation of pancreatic parenchyma or scarring can simulate a hypovascular mass [13]. Groove pancreatitis is focal, chronic pancreatitis affecting the head of the pancreas, which may result in cystic change of the adjacent duodenum and this can mimic PDAC [14]. Awareness of these entities, attention to the proper imaging technique, and correlation with symptoms and relevant lab tests can help avoid misdiagnosing these cases as tumor.

Imaging plays a key role in the staging of PDAC. Typically, this is performed with CT because CT can achieve higher spatial resolution images and is less prone to artifact compared to MRI. PDAC frequently spreads to involve the adjacent vasculature which may preclude surgical resection. Limited involvement of the adjacent arteries and veins may be treated with radiation and chemotherapy in an attempt to shrink the tumor to the point where surgical resection is possible (borderline resectable). An excellent summary of the proper imaging technique and a detailed description of the imaging findings of resectable, borderline resectable, and locally advanced PDAC was published in *Gastroenterology* in 2014 [15]. Limited involvement of adjacent vasculature (contact of superior mesenteric artery less than 180 degrees, focal distortion of superior mesenteric vein without vessel occlusion) will be deemed borderline resectable (Fig. 6). More significant tumor spread (tumor contact of celiac axis or aorta, extensive venous involvement with vessel occlusion) will be deemed locally advanced and will not

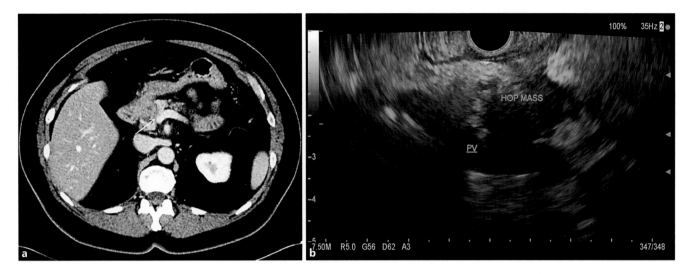

Fig. 6. Borderline resectable pancreatic cancer. **a** CT shows a hypoenhancing mass in the head of the pancreas invading the duodenum and adjacent portal vein (the arrow shows portal vein involvement). There is less than 180 degrees of vessel involvement and no venous occlusion. **b** EUS verifies the appearance of portal vein invasion.

be resected (Fig. 7). When CT is performed and interpreted correctly it has a high positive predictive value (PPV) for locally advanced tumor (89–100%) [15]. The PPV for resectable tumor is lower (45–79%) but this is because the criteria are designed to err on the side of not excluding patients who may have resectable tumor [15]. A summary of the features of resectable and locally advanced tumor according to the National Comprehensive Cancer Network (NCCN) guidelines is provided in Table 4.

Pancreatic neuroendocrine tumors deserve special attention because these tumors can be evaluated with functional imaging rather than just CT and MRI. PanNETs express high-affinity somatostatin receptors and imaging agents targeted to these receptors (for example ^{111}In pentetreotide or OctreoScan) can detect sites of PanNET [16]. The latest development in the imaging of PanNETs is the development of Gallium-68-labeled conjugated peptides to image somatostatin receptors. [68]Ga 1,4,7,10-tetraazacyclododecane-1,4,7,10-tetraacetic acid (DOTA)-octreotate (DOTATATE) is now an FDA-approved agent for imaging PanNETs. Imaging with these agents has been shown to be more sensitive and specific than imaging with ^{111}In and CT [17]. Numerous series have shown that imaging with ^{68}Ga-DOTA agents change patient management compared to imaging with OctreoScan and CT [17, 18]. As these agents become more widely available they will become the standard of care for the initial staging of patients with PanNET. Other imaging modalities will still play a role even once ^{68}Ga-DOTA imaging

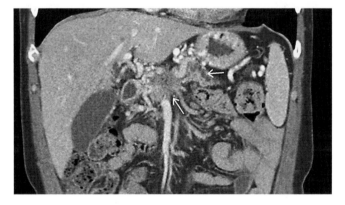

Fig. 7. Locally advanced pancreatic cancer. A coronal image from a pancreas CT scan shows a pancreatic mass (middle arrow) invading the venous confluence with occlusion and numerous collateral vessels in the upper abdomen. The arrow in the right upper quadrant shows dilation of the main pancreatic duct in the atrophic pancreatic tail.

for PanNET becomes more widespread. CT and MRI will still be useful to evaluate the response to therapy and possible disease recurrence after resection [19].

When patients are referred for endoscopic evaluation of a "pancreatic mass," there are many imaging characteristics that help narrow down the differential diagnosis of a solid mass based on the ultrasound tissue echogenicity. For a typical PDAC, the mass will be "hypoechoic" or darker than its

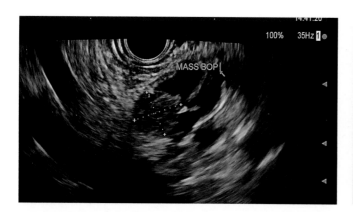

Fig. 8. Adenocarcinoma. EUS showing a small mass with downstream pancreatic ductal dilation. FNA of the mass was diagnostic for adenocarcinoma.

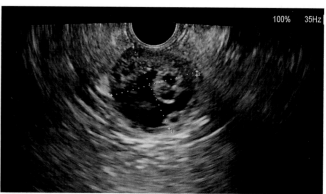

Fig. 9. Pancreatic neuroendocrine tumor, cystic. EUS showing a solid/cystic lesion in the body of the pancreas. FNA of the solid component was diagnostic for a cystic neuroendocrine tumor of the pancreas body.

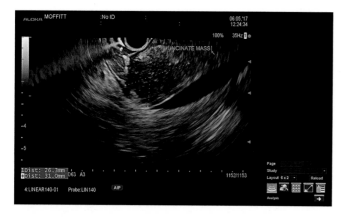

Fig. 10. Lymphoma. EUS showing a lesion in the uncinate process of the pancreas. FNA for cytology and flow cytometry revealed findings consistent with lymphoma metastasis to the pancreas.

surroundings (Fig. 8). For neuroendocrine tumors, the tumor will be well circumscribed and may have either a hypoechoic or a mixed echogenic appearance (bright and dark; Fig. 9). PanNETs are also very vascular, which can be seen when turning on the Doppler capability of the EUS scope. Metastatic malignancies are either hypoechoic or hyperechoic, and numerous lesions are typically noted (Fig. 10). A summary of the typical echogenic features is presented in Table 5.

Cystic Lesions
It can be very difficult to specifically diagnose a cystic pancreatic lesion solely on imaging characteristics. The first step

is to generate a differential diagnosis based on the imaging features of the cystic lesion. A good initial step is to classify the lesion based on its morphology as a unilocular cystic lesion, multilocular cystic lesion, or a lesion with a mixed solid/cystic appearance (Table 6).

The differential for a unilocular cystic lesion includes pseudocyst, intraductal papillary mucinous neoplasm (IPMN), and unilocular serous cystadenoma [20]. Pseudocyst should always be included in the differential of a unilocular cystic pancreatic lesion. If the patient has a history of pancreatitis the diagnosis may be unequivocal. Careful attention must be paid to evaluate for imaging signs of prior pancreatitis if there is doubt based on clinical history. Clues of prior pancreatitis include: pancreatic calcifications, atrophy of pancreatic parenchyma, and main pancreatic duct dilation and calculi [21]. Pseudocysts may communicate with the main pancreatic duct and may have a complex appearance secondary to internal blood products or necrotic debris [20]. Internal enhancement of soft tissue components should not be present in a pseudocyst and raises the possibility of a malignant cystic lesion. If nodular enhancement in a pseudocyst is seen, a pseudoaneurysm related to prior pancreatitis should also be considered [22]. Internal layering debris on T2-weighted images is a specific sign of pseudocyst but will not always be seen [23]. In indeterminate cases follow-up imaging may be useful as pseudocysts can shrink over time. Serous cystadenomas typically exhibit numerous internal septations but can manifest as a simple, unilocular cyst [24]. In these cases, a prospective diagnosis may be impossible by imaging alone. Side-branch-type IPMNs may present as a unilocular cyst. Com-

Table 5. EUS characteristics of common solid lesions of the pancreas

Type of solid mass	EUS features	Images
Adenocarcinoma	Hypoechoic, irregular borders, dilated pancreas duct	Fig. 7
Neuroendocrine tumor	Hyper- or hypoechoic, well-defined borders/solid or cystic	Fig. 8
Metastatic cancer to the pancreas	Multiple lesions, normal pancreatic duct, can be hypoechoic or hyperechoic	Fig. 9

Table 6. Cystic pancreatic masses

Unilocular	
Pseudocyst	Clinical history and imaging signs of prior pancreatitis
	Internal debris or blood products, no internal enhancement
	May shrink over time
Intraductal papillary mucinous neoplasm	Communication with main pancreatic duct
Serous cystadenoma	Can present as a single cyst
Multilocular	
Mucinous cystic neoplasm	Usually body + tail
Intraductal papillary mucinous neoplasm	Communication with the main pancreatic duct
Serous cystadenoma	Many small internal cysts
	Lobulated contour
	Central scar ± calcifications

munication to the main pancreatic duct may help make the diagnosis by imaging. However, this may be hard to demonstrate conclusively, and pseudocysts can also show this feature.

The differential for a multilocular cystic lesion includes mucinous cystic neoplasm (MCN), IPMN, and serous cystadenoma. Serous cystadenoma can be differentiated from MCN and IPMN based on its typical microcystic appearance, i.e., very numerous, small internal septations versus fewer internal septations and larger internal locules [20]. Other clues to a serous cystadenoma are external lobulations, and a central scar with or without calcifications [25] (Fig. 11). IPMN may exhibit a complex internal architecture with numerous septations. The diagnosis can be made when there is unequivocal communication with the main pancreatic duct. MCN (mucinous cystadenoma/cystadenocarcinoma) predominantly present in the body and tail of the pancreas and appear cystic with internal septations. Increasing internal complexity with thicker septations and nodularity suggests malignant degeneration.

Lesions with a mixed solid and cystic appearance include some of the cystic lesions above which exhibit malignant degeneration (IPMN, MCN) and solid pancreatic tumors with cystic or necrotic change. Common solid tumors which show this type of change are NET, SPN, PDAC, and metastases [20, 25].

CT and MRI can detect cystic lesions of the pancreas and the imaging features will help define a differential diagnosis. Unfortunately, it is difficult in many cases to make a specific diagnosis by imaging alone. For example, a recent review found CT had an accuracy of 39.0–44.7% for making a specific diagnosis of cystic pancreatic lesions [5]. Although various lesions have a typical appearance, there is significant overlap of imaging features and all of these lesions can exhibit atypical features. For example, a unilocular cyst could be a pseudocyst or unilocular serous cystadenoma. However, it could also be an IPMN or even an MCN, even though this is not a common appearance for these lesions (Fig. 12). That means the differential based on imaging includes both benign and premalignant (or malignant) lesions, an unsatisfactory situation when making a decision about patient management or follow-up.

Imaging does have more uniform success in determining if a cystic lesion is benign or malignant. For example, the previously mentioned review found a sensitivity and specificity of 36.3–71.4 and 63.9–100% for CT for determination of benign disease [5]. Other series have found accuracy in the range of 70–80% for separating benign from malignant

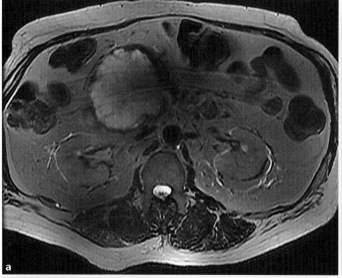

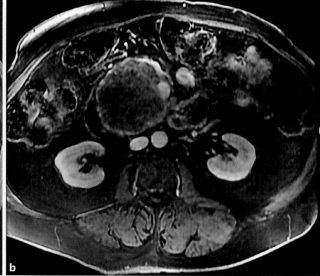

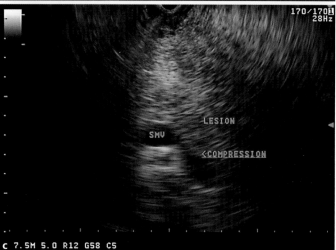

Fig. 11. Serous cystadenoma. T2-weighted (**a**) and postcontrast (**b**) MRI images show a lesion in the head of the pancreas. The lesion is cystic based on the T2-weighted image, and numerous very small enhancing septations are seen. The characteristic lobulations of serous cystadenoma are best seen on the T2-weighted image. **c** By EUS the very small internal septations mimic a solid mass.

Fig. 12. Cystic pancreatic lesion – IPMN. **a** A T2-weighted image from an MRI shows a cyst in the body of the pancreas with a thin internal septation. **b** EUS shows the lesion and the internal septation. The differential based on the appearance could be an IPMN, MCN, pseudocyst, oligocystic serous cystadenoma, and even cystic PanNET. Other images appeared to show a communication with the main pancreatic duct and aspiration yielded mucin, confirming a pancreatic IPMN.

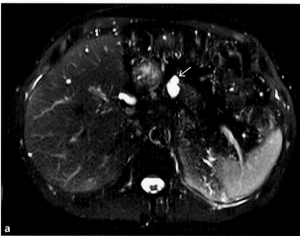

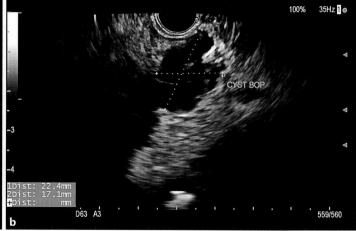

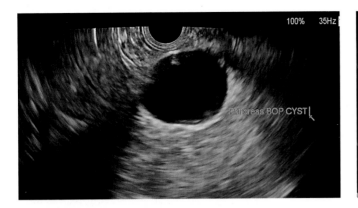

Fig. 13. EUS showing a unilocular cyst without pancreatic ductal communication. FNA revealed an MCN of the pancreas body.

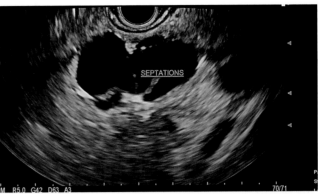

Fig. 14. Incidental cystic lesion found on a CT scan which on EUS revealed a septated and tortuous cystic lesion consistent with a side-branch IPMN.

cystic lesions by CT [26]. MRI can perform even better, with various series showing sensitivity, specificity, and accuracy surpassing CT [26]. For example, one series found that MRI had an accuracy of 85–91% for establishing benign lesions [27]. MRI also shows accuracy close to 100% for establishing lesion communication with the main pancreatic duct [5]. Although MRI, especially when MRCP sequences are included, offers an improved evaluation of cystic pancreatic lesions, research has suggested CT provides a comparable evaluation with regards to clinical decision making [28]. There are numerous imaging features which may assist in the evaluation of the malignant potential of a cystic pancreatic lesion. One of the features most concerning for malignancy is an enhancing mural nodule within a cystic lesion [26, 29, 30]. CT and MRI can diagnose a mural nodule based on postcontrast enhancement, but care must be taken to avoid misdiagnosing a hematoma, calcification, or inspissated mucin as a mural nodule. Other features shown to correlate with malignancy are dilation of the common bile duct, increasing lesion complexity, and the presence of multiple cystic lesions [29, 31–33]. CT and MRI can detect these features with high sensitivity and accuracy, which explains the published good results for distinguishing benign from malignant cystic lesions. However, accurate identification of these features does not guarantee a successful classification. As the authors of one series point out, two lesions which were unilocular and smaller than 1 cm in size showed frank malignancy at pathologic evaluation [34].

EUS is an extremely valuable imaging modality for the evaluation of pancreatic cystic lesions. Although, as mentioned earlier, certain cysts have very characteristic imaging

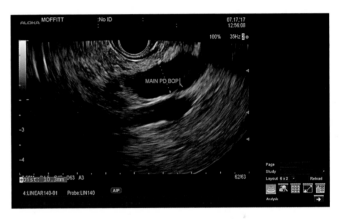

Fig. 15. EUS of the head of the pancreas revealed a markedly dilated main pancreatic duct in the body of the pancreas.

findings, EUS cannot only confirm these imaging findings, but in certain situations also be used to perform FNA to confirm or exclude a certain diagnosis, which in many instances can change the management of the patient. EUS can also detect small nodules in cysts, septations, or a thickened cyst wall that may not be readily apparent on other imaging modalities, including CT scan or MRI. Although it can be difficult for EUS to distinguish a mural nodule from a mucus clump in a side branch IPMN, there are certain EUS characteristic findings that can help distinguish one from the other, including the vascularity of contrast enhancement and the echogenicity characteristics of the nodule. Nodules that lack vascularity on EUS Doppler flow and have shadow characteristics are more consistent with mucus plugs,

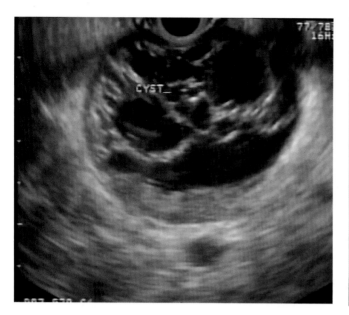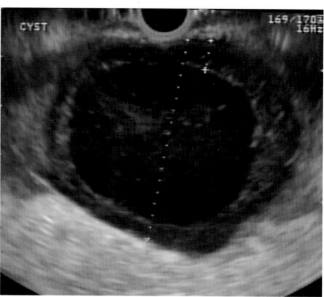

Fig. 16. EUS showing a cystic lesion with a honeycomb appearance that is multiseptated consistent with a serous cystadenoma of the body of the pancreas.

Fig. 17. EUS in a patient with history of pancreatitis revealed a cyst in the body of the pancreas that is unilocular with a thickened wall and internal debris. FNA for cytology and CEA and amylase were consistent with a pseudocyst of the pancreas.

Table 7. EUS characteristics of cystic lesions of the pancreas

Cyst	EUS features	Management	Images
MCN	Unilocular, macrocystic, anechoic, few septations, PD normal	Surgery	Fig. 13
SB-IPMN (low-risk)	Normal main PD, dilated branch of the PD cysts <3 cm	MRI/MRCP imaging surveillance	Fig. 14
SB-IPMN (high-risk)	Normal main PD, cystic structures >3 cm, mural nodules	Surgery	
Main-duct IPMN	Dilated main PD >7 mm	Surgery	Fig. 15
Serous cystadenoma	Multiseptated, microcystic, honeycomb appearance, central calcification	Benign – no treatment unless growing and causing symptoms	Fig. 16
Pseudocyst	Thick-walled, unilocular, debris-filled, history of pancreatitis	Cyst drainage if symptomatic or concern for infection	Fig. 17

PD, pancreatic duct.

whereas vascular-enhancing nodules that are hypoechoic and do not shadow are more consistent with true mural nodules. Distinguishing between the two is of paramount importance as a nodule is considered a high-risk feature that warrants surgical resection, whereas a mucus clump is a benign finding. EUS imaging characteristics of cystic lesions of the pancreas are summarized in Table 7 and illustrated in Figures 13–17.

Disclosure Statement

The authors have no conflicts of interest to disclose.

References

1 Morgan D, Stanley R: The pancreas; in Lee J, Sagel S, Stanley R, Heiken J (eds): Computed Body Tomography with MRI Correlation. Philadelphia: Lippincott, Williams and Wilkins, 2006, pp 1007–1100.

2 Boland G, Maiiey ME, Saez M, Fernandez-del-castillo C, Warshaw AL, Mueller PR: Pancreatic-phase versus portal vein-phase helical CT of the pancreas. Am J Roentgenol 1999;172:605–608.

3 Altun E, Elias J, Armao D, Vachiranubhap B, Semelka R: Pancreas; in Semelka R (ed): Abdominal-Pelvic MRI, ed 3. Hoboken, Wiley-Blackwell, 2010, pp 535–676.

4 Vitellas KM, Keogan MT, Spritzer CE, Nelson RC: MR cholangiopancreatography of bile and pancreatic duct abnormalities with emphasis on the single-shot fast spin-echo technique. Radiographics 2013;20:939–957.

5 Jones MJ, Buchanan AS, Neal CP, Dennison AR, Metcalfe MS, Garcea G: Imaging of indeterminate pancreatic cystic lesions: a systematic review. Pancreatology 2013;13:436–442.

6 Federle M: EXPERTddx: Abdomen, ed 1. Salt Lake City, Amirsys, 2009.

7 Low G, Panu A, Millo N, Leen E: Multimodality imaging of neoplastic and nonneoplastic solid lesions of the pancreas. Radiographics 2011;31:993–1015.

8 Lee WK, Lau EWF, Duddalwar VA, Stanley AJ, Ho YY: Abdominal manifestations of extranodal lymphoma: spectrum of imaging findings. Am J Roentgenol 2008;191:198–206.

9 Merkle EM, Bender GN, Brambs HJ: Imaging findings in pancreatic lymphoma: differential aspects. Am J Roentgenol 2000;174:671–675.

10 Coakley FV, Hanley-Knutson K, Mongan J, Barajas R, Bucknor M, Qayyum A: Pancreatic imaging mimics: part 1, imaging mimics of pancreatic adenocarcinoma. Am J Roentgenol 2012;199:301–308.

11 Choi JY, Kim MJ, Kim JH, Kim SH, Lim JS, Oh YT, Chung JJ, Yoo HS, Lee JT, Kim KW: Solid pseudopapillary tumor of the pancreas: typical and atypical manifestations. Am J Roentgenol 2006;187:178–186.

12 Morse B, Centeno B, Vignesh S: Autoimmune pancreatitis: updated concepts of a challenging diagnosis. Am J Med 2014;127:1010.e1–9.

13 Muhi A, Ichikawa T, Motosugi U, Sou H, Sano K, Tsukamoto T, Fatima Z, Araki T: Mass-forming autoimmune pancreatitis and pancreatic carcinoma: differential diagnosis on the basis of computed tomography and magnetic resonance cholangiopancreatography, and diffusion-weighted imaging findings. J Magn Reson Imaging 2012;3:827–836.

14 Miller F, Keppke A, Wadhwa A, Ly J, Dalal K, Kamler V: MRI of pancreatitis and its complications: part 2, chronic pancreatitis. Am J Roentgenol 2004;183:1645–1652.

15 Al-Hawary MM, Francis IR, Chari ST, Fishman EK, Hough DM, Lu DS, Macari M, Megibow AJ, Miller FH, Mortele KJ, Merchant NB, Minter RM, Tamm EP, Sahani DV, Simeone DM: Pancreatic ductal adenocarcinoma radiology reporting template: consensus statement of the society of abdominal radiology and the American Pancreatic Association. Gastroenterology 2014;146:291–304.e1.

16 De Herde WW: Functional localisation and scintigraphy in neuroendocrine tumours of the gastrointestinal tract and pancreas (GEP-NETs). Eur J Endocrinol 2014;170:R173–R183.

17 Sadowski SM, Neychev V, Millo C, Shih J, Nilubol N, Herscovitch P, Pacak K, Marx SJ, Kebebew E: Prospective study of ^{68}Ga-DOTATATE positron emission tomography/computed tomography for detecting gastro-entero-pancreatic neuroendocrine tumors and unknown primary sites. J Clin Oncol 2016;34:588–597.

18 Deppen SA, Liu E, Blume JD, Clanton J, Shi C, Jones-Jackson LB, Lakhani V, Baum R, Berlin J, Smith G, Graham M, Sandler M, Delbeke D, Walker RC: Safety and efficacy of ^{68}Ga-DOTATATE PET/CT for diagnosis, staging and treatment management of neuroendocrine tumors. J Nucl Med 2016;57:708–715.

19 Kim K, Krajewski K, Nishino M, Jagannathan J, Shinagare A, Tirumani S, Ramaiya N: Update on the management of gastroenteropancreatic neuroendocrine tumors with emphasis on the role of imaging. Am J Roentgenol 2014;201:811–824.

20 Sahani DV, Kadavigere R, Saokar A, Fernandez-del Castillo C, Brugge WR, Hahn PF: Cystic pancreatic lesions: a simple imaging-based classification system for guiding management. Radiographics 2005;25:1471–1484.

21 Sahani DV, Miller JC, Fernàndez del Castillo C, Brugge WR, Thrall JH, Lee SI: Cystic pancreatic lesions: classification and management. J Am Coll Radiol 2009;6:376–380.

22 Hughey M, Taffel M, Zeman RK, Patel S, Hill MC: The diagnostic challenge of the sequelae of acute pancreatitis on CT imaging: a pictorial essay. Abdom Radiol 2017;42:1199–1209.

23 Macari M, Finn ME, Bennett GL, Cho KC, Newman E, Hajdu CH, Babb JS: Differentiating pancreatic cystic neoplasms from pancreatic pseudocysts at MR imaging: value of perceived internal debris. Radiology 2009;251:77–84.

24 Cohen-Scali F, Vilgrain V, Brancatelli G, Hammel P, Vullierme M-P, Sauvanet A, Menu Y: Discrimination of unilocular macrocystic serous cystadenoma from pancreatic pseudocyst and mucinous cystadenoma with CT: initial observations. Radiology 2003;228:727–733.

25 Kalb B, Sarmiento JM, Kooby D, Adsay NV, Martin DR: MR imaging of cystic lesions of the pancreas. Radiographics 2009;29:1749–1765.

26 Dahani DV, Kambadakone A, MacAri M, Takahashi N, Chari S, Fernandez-Del Castillo C: Diagnosis and management of cystic pancreatic lesions. Am J Roentgenol 2013;200:343–354.

27 Visser BC, Yeh BM, Qayyum A, Way LW, McCulloch CE, Coakley FV: Characterization of cystic pancreatic masses: relative accuracy of CT and MRI. Am J Roentgenol 2007;89:648–656.

28 Sainani NI, Saokar A, Deshpande V, Fernandez-del Castillo C, Hahn P, Sahani DV: Comparative performance of MDCT and MRI with MR cholangiopancreatography in characterizing small pancreatic cysts. Am J Roentgenol 2009;193:722–731.

29 Kim KW, Park SH, Pyo J, Yoon SH, Byun JH, Lee M-G, Krajewski KM, Ramaiya NH: Imaging features to distinguish malignant and benign branch-duct type intraductal papillary mucinous neoplasms of the pancreas: a meta-analysis. Ann Surg 2014;259:72–81.

30 Kawamoto S, Horton KM, Lawler LP, Hruban RH, Fishman EK: Intraductal papillary mucinous neoplasm of the pancreas: can benign lesions be differentiated from malignant lesions with multidetector CT? Radiographics 2005;25:1451–1470.

31 Paroder V, Flusberg M, Kobi M, Rozenblit AM, Chernyak V: Pancreatic cysts: what imaging characteristics are associated with development of pancreatic ductal adenocarcinoma? Eur J Radiol 2016;85:1622–1626.

32 Kawamoto S, Lawler LP, Horton KM, Eng J, Hruban RH, Fishman EK: MDCT of intraductal papillary mucinous neoplasm of the pancreas: evaluation of features predictive of invasive carcinoma. Am J Roentgenol 2006;186:687–695.

33 Strauss A, Birdsey M, Fritz S, Schwarz-Bundy BD, Bergmann F, Hackert T, Kauczor H-U, Grenacher L, Klauss M: Intraductal papillary mucinous neoplasms of the pancreas: radiological predictors of malignant transformation and the introduction of bile duct dilation to current guidelines. Br J Radiol 2016;89:1061.

34 Visser BC, Yeh BM, Qayyum A, Way LW, McCulloch CE, Coakley FV: Characterization of cystic pancreatic masses: relative accuracy of CT and MRI. Am J Roentgenol 2007;189:648–656.

Prof. Jason Klapman
Moffitt Cancer Center
12902 USF Magnolia Drive
Tampa, FL 33612 (USA)
jason.klapman@moffitt.org

Chapter 4

Published online: September 29, 2020

Centeno BA, Dhillon J (eds): Pancreatic Tumors. Monogr Clin Cytol. Basel, Karger, 2020, vol 26, pp 34–41 (DOI:10.1159/000455733)

Normal Components and Contaminants

Jasreman Dhillon[a, b]

[a]Department of Anatomic Pathology, Moffitt Cancer Center, Tampa, FL, USA; [b]Department of Oncologic Sciences and Pathology, University of South Florida, Tampa, FL, USA

Abstract

The pancreas is a retroperitoneal organ located in the duodenal loop with the posterior wall of the stomach overlying it and the left lobe of the liver lying anteriorly to it. Tissues from these organs, in addition to the lesion of interest within the pancreas, may be sampled during fine-needle aspiration (FNA) procedures. Therefore, it is important to recognize the cytology of normal benign components of the pancreas and potential contaminants in order to render a correct diagnosis and avoid pitfalls. Normal components of the pancreas include ductal epithelial cells, acinar cells, and islet cells. In addition to the normal pancreatic cells, it is not uncommon to encounter epithelial cells from the duodenal and gastric mucosa with endoscopic ultrasound-guided fine-needle aspiration. It is important to recognize these cells as benign and to distinguish them from a well-differentiated pancreatic adenocarcinoma. Besides these, mesothelial cells and hepatocytes and bile duct cells from the liver may be sampled as well. Here, the cytological features of normal components and contaminants are described in detail.

© 2020 S. Karger AG, Basel

Normal Anatomy

The pancreas is a retroperitoneal organ that is located at the level of the 2nd and 3rd lumbar vertebrae. It extends from the duodenal loop across the midline towards the spleen on the left side [1]. The pancreas is composed of four anatomic regions that are not sharply demarcated from one another: the head, neck, body, and tail. The head of the pancreas is attached to the 2nd and 3rd portions of the duodenum. The neck of the gland lies inferior to the pylorus. The posterior wall of the stomach overlies the body and the proximal jejunum passes inferior to the body, immediately distal to the ligament of Treitz. The distal portion of the common bile duct passes through the posterior superior head of the pancreas and enters the duodenum at the ampulla of Vater. The left lobe of the liver lies anterior to the head. The posterior aspect of the body of the pancreas lies in close approximation to the left adrenal gland and kidney. Because of the proximity of the pancreas to several organs, tissue from these organs may be inadvertently sampled during a fine-needle aspiration procedure. Hence, it is important to identify the location of the mass in the pancreas and be able to identify normal tissue cytology under the microscope.

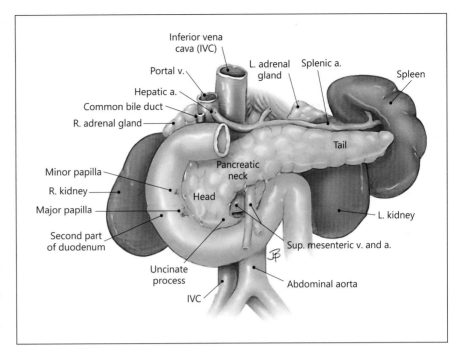

Fig. 1. Anatomic relationship of the pancreas with surrounding organs and structures. a, artery; l, left; r, right; v, vein. Artwork by Jennifer Parsons Brumbaugh. Reproduced with permission from the American Registry of Pathology, Washington [13], in collaboration with the Armed Forces Institute of Pathology, Washington.

The uncinate process of the pancreas passes behind the neck of the pancreas and the superior mesenteric vessels. The neck of the pancreas rests anterior to the mesenteric vessels (Fig. 1). These vessels form a groove in the posterior aspect of the neck and on the anterior surface of the uncinate process. The body of the pancreas is present anterior to the aorta and extends up to the left border of the aorta. The tail of the pancreas is present in close proximity to the splenic vessels within the splenorenal ligament.

The pancreas is composed of exocrine and endocrine components that are arranged in lobules which are separated by connective tissue septa (Fig. 2). The lobules are composed of acini and ducts and with scattered islets of Langerhans.

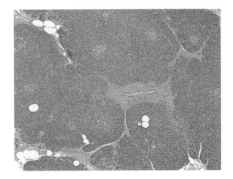

Fig. 2. Histology of the normal pancreas. The normal pancreas shows a lobular architecture separated by fibrous bands. The majority is composed of acinar cells with a few islets and ductal cells. HE stain.

Normal Pancreatic Components

Ductal Cells

The ductal system within the lobules consists of numerous intercalated ducts that fuse to form intralobular ducts (Fig. 3a). These ducts are lined by small flat to cuboidal cells with pale or lightly eosinophilic cytoplasm and oval central nuclei. Intralobular ducts come together to form interlobular ducts that are surrounded by a variably thick rim of dense fibrous tissue (Fig. 3b). The cells tend to become low columnar with relatively more cytoplasm as the ducts enlarge. The nuclei of the larger ducts are round and basally located with apical cytoplasmic clearing, reflecting mucin deposition. However, complete replacement of the cytoplasm by mucin is indicative of the earliest step in neoplastic transformation, pancreatic intraepithelial neoplasia grade 1.

Cytology

Ductal epithelial cells of the pancreas are cuboidal to columnar and may be pseudostratified. The cells are arranged in

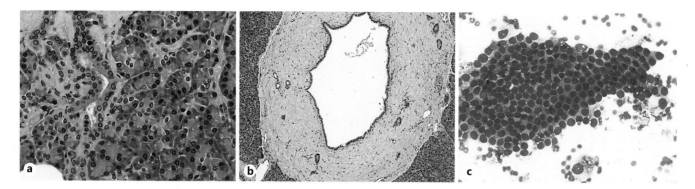

Fig. 3. Normal ducts. **a** Intercalated ducts lined by cuboidal cells, a scant amount of cytoplasm and round nuclei. HE stain, ×40. **b** Interlobular ducts and surrounding fibrotic tissue. HE stain. **c** Benign ductal epithelial cells present in a honeycombed pattern. Diff-Quik stain.

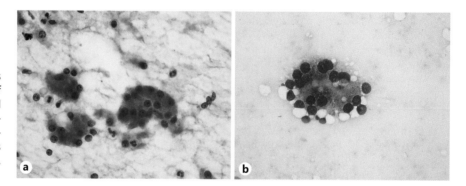

Fig. 4. a Acinar cells. Groups of acinar cells with a moderate to abundant amount of granular cytoplasm and basally located round nuclei with prominent nucleoli. Papanicolaou stain. **b** Acinar cells showing a moderate amount of cytoplasm with granules and round nuclei with prominent nucleoli. Diff-Quik stain.

2-dimensional sheets, strips, and clusters, and exhibit honeycombing [2] (Fig. 3c). The epithelial clusters may exhibit peripheral palisading where the nuclei are basally located. The nuclei may be centrally located as well and be round to oval with smooth membranes. A key point is that normal ductal epithelium lacks cytoplasmic mucin, so ductal/glandular-type cells with cytoplasm showing mucinous metaplasia are not normal.

Key Cytological Features
- Cuboidal to columnar epithelial cells
- Flat, 2-dimensional, honeycomb sheets or peripherally palisading cells with basally located nuclei
- Moderate amount of non-mucinous cytoplasm
- Round to oval nuclei with smooth membranes

Acinar Cells
The acinar cells are the main exocrine secretory component of the gland, and normal pancreas is composed mainly of acinar cells. On microscopic examination, the acini are tightly packed, consisting of spherically arranged individual acinar cells. Acinar cells contain abundant granular eosinophilic cytoplasm in the apical aspect and basophilic basal cytoplasm [3]. The eosinophilia of the apical cytoplasm is due to the accumulation of numerous zymogen granules. The basophilia of the basal cytoplasm is due to a high concentration of ribonucleoproteins in the rough endoplasmic reticulum. The nuclei are also basally located, round, with prominent nucleoli.

Cytology
Acinar cells are the most common of the benign pancreatic cells aspirated. These cells are arranged in small, tightly cohesive, ball-like 3-dimensional or circular cell clusters or may be present singly [2, 4]. Acinar cell clusters do not usually have central lumina. The individual cells are pyramidal or triangular in shape and have a moderate to abundant amount of cytoplasm which is granulated or exhibits microvacuoles. These cells contain numerous intracytoplasmic zymogen granules. Zymogen granules stain positively with periodic acid-Schiff stain with diastase (dPAS) pretreatment, and appear as negative imprints on air-dried, Romanowsky-stained smears. The nuclei are round to oval

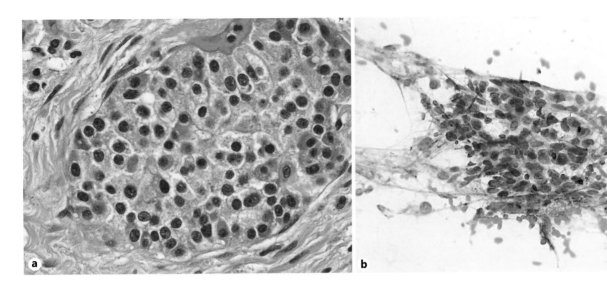

Fig. 5. Islet cells. **a** Islet cells with round nuclei and moderate amount of pale cytoplasm. HE stain. **b** Cluster of islet cells with monomorphic nuclei with a salt and pepper chromatin pattern. Papanicolaou stain.

with prominent nucleoli and are present either towards the base of the cell or are centrally located (Fig. 4a, b).

Key Cytological Features
- Small, tightly cohesive, ball-like 3-dimensional cellular clusters lacking a lumen
- Pyramidal or triangular-shaped cells with moderate to abundant granular cytoplasm
- Round to oval nuclei with prominent nucleoli
- Cytoplasmic granules, demonstrable with dPAS or else appearing as negative images on Romanowsky-stained smears

Islet Cells
The endocrine component of the pancreas constitutes 1–2% of the volume of the attached adult gland [5]. The vast majority of endocrine cells are found in the islets of Langerhans that are more numerous in the tail of the pancreas. The islets are compact, round to oval structures containing endocrine cells. The individual endocrine cells have round nuclei with stippled chromatin and inconspicuous nucleoli. A moderate amount of pale and amphophilic cytoplasm is present (Fig. 5a). Mitotic figures are rarely encountered in normal islets [6]. The major peptides produced by islet cells are insulin, glucagon, somatostatin, and pancreatic polypeptide.

Cytology
Islet cells are rarely detected in aspirates of normal pancreas. They are usually present in cases of pancreatic atrophy where the islet cells predominate. They are present in small organoid clusters or loose aggregates and form small groups. The cells are monomorphic, have round nuclei and smooth nuclear membranes with a salt and pepper stippled chromatin pattern. The islet cells have a minimal amount of fragile, wispy amphophilic cytoplasm which is often stripped away on smears resulting in the presence of naked nuclei [2] (Fig. 5b).

Key Cytological Features
- Small groups of loose aggregates of monomorphic cells
- Variable amount of amphophilic cytoplasm
- Round nuclei with stippled chromatin
- Presence of naked nuclei in the background

Gastrointestinal Contaminant

Pancreatic lesions, depending on their location, are sampled either through the stomach or the duodenum, leading to the presence of benign gastric or duodenal epithelial cells in the aspirate. Rarely squamous epithelial cells from the oral cavity or the esophagus are present on smears as contaminants.

Gastric Contaminant
The gastric mucosa is composed of tall, columnar, mucous-secreting epithelium which is the same throughout all the mucosal zones of the stomach. It is the gastric glands, present at the base of the pits, which are different types in the

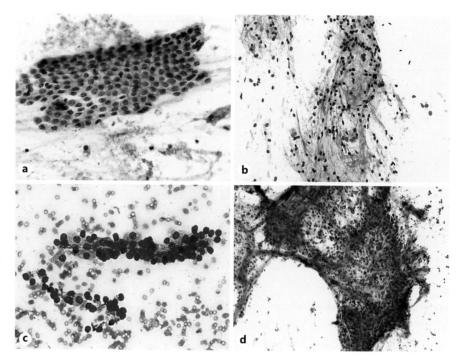

Fig. 6. Gastric contaminant. **a** Cytology of normal foveolar cells with mild degenerative changes such as nuclear grooves and nuclear contour irregularity. Papanicolaou stain. **b** Stripped nuclei with degenerative changes admixed with mucin. Diff-Quik stain. **c** Fundic mucosa with parietal and chief cells. Diff-Quik stain. **d** Lamina propria composed of fibrotic tissue with small, thin-walled blood vessels. Papanicolaou stain.

different mucosal zones. The surface epithelial cells are tall, columnar, and have basally situated nuclei containing inconspicuous nucleoli. The cytoplasm is almost entirely filled with mucus. Gastric fundic mucosa has chief cells and parietal cells, whereas pyloric mucosa contains pyloric glands that have a bubbly and foamy cytoplasm which resemble Brunner's glands of the duodenum.

Special stain PAS/Alcian blue stains the neutral mucin magenta, acid mucin light blue, and combinations purple. In the normal stomach, mucus secreted by the columnar cells is neutral and is PAS positive and negative for Alcian blue. The main mucins expressed in the stomach are MUC1 (membrane bound) and MUC5AC and MUC6 (secreted) [7]. MUC5AC forms the bulk of the mucous and is secreted by the surface foveolar cells. MUC6 is secreted by the neck and gland cells. Gastric contaminant epithelial cells show fine punctate perinuclear staining with B72.3 and strongly label for CD10 [8, 9].

Cytology

Gastric epithelial cells have mucin-containing cells that are admixed with the benign epithelium. The mucin is apical in gastric epithelium and in cases of intestinal metaplasia where goblet cells are present [2]. The benign gastric epithelial cells are present in flat, monolayered sheets with few scattered single cells in the background. The nuclei are uniform and round, with smooth nuclear contours and are evenly spaced giving a honeycomb appearance to the sheet of cells (Fig. 6a). Nucleoli are absent. The background is usually clean with the presence of mucin. Stripped nuclei with degenerative changes associated with mucin are a frequent pattern (Fig. 6b). Aspirates through the fundus may pick up gastric glands and show both parietal and chief cells (Fig. 6c). Lamina propria may be aspirated with the epithelium (Fig. 6d).

Key Cytological Features

- Flat, monolayered sheets of apical mucin containing columnar cells
- Uniform, round nuclei with inconspicuous nucleoli
- Stripped nuclei with grooves and degenerative changes in a mucinous background
- Parietal cells and chief cells
- Clean background with the presence of mucin

Duodenal Contaminant

The duodenum has a villous mucosal architecture that is lined by goblet cells and tall columnar absorptive cells. Goblet cells contain mucin that is Alcian blue and PAS positive. Brunner's glands are lobular collections of tubuloalveolar glands that are submucosal in location and are a distinctive feature of the duodenum (Fig. 7a). Brunner's glands are lined

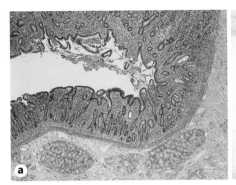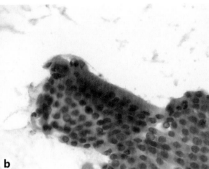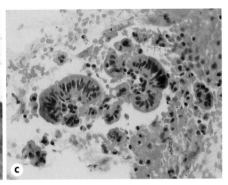

Fig. 7. Duodenal mucosa. **a** Normal histology of the duodenum with goblet cells and Brunner's glands. HE stain. **b** Cytology of normal duodenal epithelial cells with a microvillous border. Papanicolaou stain. **c** Cell block section of normal duodenal epithelial cells showing eneterocytes with a microvillous brush border. HE stain.

by cuboidal to columnar cells with pale, uniform cytoplasm and an oval, basally located nucleus. The cytoplasm contains PAS and diastase-resistant positive mucin. The absorptive cells, or enterocytes, have a microvillous brush border. Immunohistochemical studies will show expression for MUC2 in the goblet cells and for CDX2 in the entire epithelium.

Cytology

Goblet cells are abundant in duodenal epithelium. The benign duodenal epithelial cells are present in flat, monolayered sheets with few scattered single goblet cells (Fig. 7c). The duodenal non-goblet epithelial cells have a dense, non-vacuolated cytoplasm and usually have a brush border at the luminal edges (Fig. 7b) [8, 10]. The nuclei in duodenal epithelia are uniform and round, with smooth nuclear contours and are evenly spaced giving a honeycomb appearance to the sheet of cells. Nucleoli may be present in the duodenal epithelium [2]. The background is usually clean with the presence of mucin. Brunner's glands are present in loose clusters of relatively large cells that have a low nuclear-to-cytoplasmic ratio due to the presence of abundant cytoplasm. The cytoplasm is fragile, clear, and finely vacuolated. The nuclei are uniform, small, and round, with inconspicuous nucleoli and are eccentrically placed.

Key Cytological Features

- Flat, monolayered sheets of cells containing goblet cells and infiltrated by lymphocytes
- Presence of a brush border at the luminal edges of the enterocytes
- Uniform, round nuclei with inconspicuous nucleoli
- Brunner's glands composed of large cells containing abundant clear and finely vacuolated cytoplasm

Squamous Cell Contaminant

Squamous cells from either the oral cavity or the esophagus can be the source of squamous cell contamination in the pancreatic aspirations. The squamous cells are usually superficial and mature, with a centrally located round nucleus. Oropharyngeal contamination has a mixed population of bacteria in addition to the mature squamous cells and many bacteria are seen adherent to the surface of the epithelial cells without the presence of neutrophils.

Cytology

The superficial squamous cells are eosinophilic polygonal-shaped cells with a centrally placed pyknotic nucleus. Intermediate squamous cells typically stain basophilic with Papanicolaou stain. There is a centrally placed nucleus with vesicular, finely dispersed granular chromatin (Fig. 8).

Key Cytological Features

- Polygonal eosinophilic cells with a central pyknotic nucleus
- Intermediate basophilic cells with a vesicular and finely dispersed chromatin
- Mixed population of bacteria without the presence of neutrophils

Mesothelial Contaminant

Overview

The mesothelium is the layer of cells that lines the serous membranes of the peritoneum. Mesothelial cells have an abundant, clear cytoplasm and well-defined cell borders.

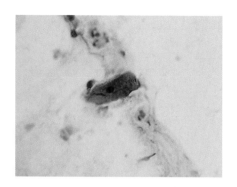

Fig. 8. Squamous cells. Oropharyngeal contamination with bacteria adherent to a mature squamous cell. Papanicolaou stain.

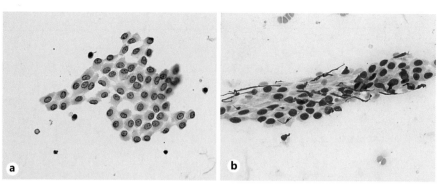

Fig. 9. Mesothelial cells. **a, b** Sheets of benign mesothelial cells with well-defined cytoplasmic borders. Papanicolaou and Diff-Quik stain.

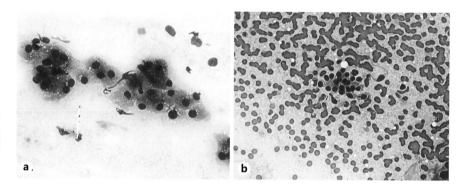

Fig. 10. Liver contaminant. **a** Benign hepatocytes with round centrally placed nuclei and a moderate amount of cytoplasm containing bile pigment. Diff-Quik stain. **b** A cluster of cuboidal bile duct epithelial cells with round nuclei and scant cytoplasm. Diff-Quik stain.

The nuclei are small, centrally placed, and without a nucleolus. In reactive processes, nucleoli may become prominent.

Cytology
Mesothelial cells may be inadvertently sampled depending on the approach. Mesothelial cells are present as honeycomb sheets of evenly spaced, uniform cells with abundant cytoplasm (Fig. 9a, b). There are narrow gaps or windows present within adjoining cells due to the presence of the microvilli. The nuclei are small and round, with the presence of discrete nucleoli [11].

Key Cytological Features
• Honeycomb sheets of evenly spaced uniform cells with intercytoplasmic windows
• Small, round nuclei

Liver Contaminant

Hepatocytes
The liver is composed of parenchymal, interstitial, vascular, and ductal elements. The hepatocytes are arranged in plates one cell layer thick in adults. Hepatocytes are polygonal cells with an abundant amount of cytoplasm, which is eosinophilic. Lipofuscin, hemosiderin, and bile pigments may be present in varying amounts in the cytoplasm. Most of the hepatocytes have a single, centrally located round nucleus with a prominent nucleolus. Each portal tract contains a bile duct and ductules, a hepatic artery branch, a portal vein branch, and lymphatic channels embedded in connective tissue.

Cytology
Occasionally, normal liver can be sampled during the aspiration procedure. Aspirates of normal liver are predominantly composed of hepatocytes and scattered bile duct epithelial cells. The hepatocytes can be arranged singly, in 2-di-

mensional small- to large-sized clusters and 2- to 3-cell-layer-thick trabeculae [12]. The hepatocytes are polygonal to round cells with an abundant cytoplasm, which may be dense granular to vacuolated due to the presence of lipid or glycogen (Fig. 10a). Hepatocytes may contain pigments like lipofuscin, bile, or hemosiderin within the cytoplasm. There is usually a single nucleus with a prominent nucleolus. However, binucleated cells and cells with intranuclear inclusions are not uncommon.

Key Cytological Features
- Polygonal cells with an abundant eosinophilic cytoplasm
- Cytoplasm may contain pigments
- Usually a centrally placed, round nucleus with prominent nucleolus

Bile Duct Cells
The larger intrahepatic bile ducts are lined by tall columnar epithelial cells that contain light eosinophilic cytoplasm. The smaller bile ducts are lined by cuboidal to low columnar cells.

The epithelial cells contain a single, basally situated oval nucleus. Bile ducts are present within the portal tracts and are always accompanied by a portal vein and a hepatic artery.

Cytology
Bile duct epithelial cells are cuboidal to columnar and form monolayered honeycomb sheets. Nuclei are small and round, with a condensed nuclear chromatin and inconspicuous nucleoli [12]. A scant amount of cytoplasm is present (Fig. 10b).

Key Cytological Features
- Honeycomb sheets of cuboidal to columnar epithelial cells with basally located nuclei
- Scant cytoplasm

Disclosure Statement

The author has no conflicts of interest to report.

References

1 Fawcett DW: Bloom and Fawcett. A textbook of histology, ed 12. New York, Chapman and Hall, 1994.
2 Layfield LJ, Jarboe EA: Cytopathology of the pancreas: neoplastic and nonneoplastic entities. Ann Diagn Pathol 2010;14:140–151.
3 Klimstra DS, Sternberg SS: Histology for Pathologists, ed 2. Philadelphia, Lippincott, Williams and Wilkins, 1997, pp 613–647.
4 Leiman G: My approach to pancreatic fine needle aspiration. J Clin Pathol 2007;60:43–49.
5 Williams JA, Goldfine ID: The insulin-acinar relationship; in Go VLW, Gardner JD, Brooks FP, Lebenthal E, DiMagno EP, Scheele GA (eds): The Exocrine Pancreas. Biology, Pathobiology, and Diseases. New York, Raven, 1986, pp 347–360.
6 LeCompte PM, Merriam JC: Mitotic figures and enlarged nuclei in the islands of Langerhans in man. Diabetes 1962;11:35–39.
7 Niv Y: *H. pylori*/NSAID – negative peptic ulcer – the mucin theory. Med Hypotheses 2010;75: 433–435.
8 Nawgiri RS, Nagle JA, Wilbur DC, Pitman MB: Cytomorphology and B72.3 labeling of benign and malignant ductal epithelium in pancreatic lesions compared to gastrointestinal epithelium. Diagn Cytopathol 2007;35:300–305.
9 Vigliar E, Troncone G, Bracale U, Iaccarino A, Napolitano V, Bellevicine C: CD10 is useful to identify gastrointestinal contamination in endoscopic ultrasound-guided fine needle aspiration (EUS-FNA) cytology from pancreatic ductal adenocarcinoma. Cytopathology 2015;26:83–87.
10 Nagle JA, Wilbur DC, Pitman MB: Cytomorphology of gastric and duodenal epithelium and reactivity to B72.3: a baseline for comparison to pancreatic lesions aspirated by EUS-FNAB. Diagn Cytopathol 2005;33:381–386.
11 Sidawy MK, Ali SZ: Fine Needle Aspiration Cytology. Amsterdam, Elsevier, 2007, p 159.
12 Chhieng DC: Fine needle aspiration biopsy of liver – an update. World J Surg Oncol 2004;2:5.
13 Hruban RH, Pitman MB, Klimstra DS: AFIP Atlas of Tumor Pathology Series 4: Tumors of the Pancreas. Washington, American Registry of Pathology, 2007.

Dr. Jasreman Dhillon
Moffitt Cancer Center
12902 USF Magnolia Drive
Tampa, FL 33612 (USA)
jasreman.dhillon@moffitt.org

Published online: September 29, 2020

Centeno BA, Dhillon J (eds): Pancreatic Tumors. Monogr Clin Cytol. Basel, Karger, 2020, vol 26, pp 42–52 (DOI:10.1159/000455734)

Non-Neoplastic Masses of the Pancreas

Barbara A. Centeno[a, b]   Sarah C. Thomas[c]

[a]Department of Pathology, Moffitt Cancer Center, Tampa, FL, USA; [b]Department of Oncologic Sciences, Morsani College of Medicine, University of South Florida, Tampa, FL, USA; [c]Office of Chief Medical Examiner, New York, NY, USA

Abstract

Benign non-neoplastic solid lesions of the pancreas are comprised of several separate entities, with their diagnostic identification best performed in correlation with the radiographic and clinical features. These include all of the pancreatitides, intrapancreatic spleen, and a few other rare entities. Preoperative imaging may suggest the correct diagnosis, but occasionally the preoperative imaging findings may be misleading because they overlap with those of pancreatic neoplasms. Masses associated with typical pancreatitides are rarely sampled due to their distinct clinical picture and relative frequency; however, the uncommon variants of pancreatitis may also present as mass lesions mimicking malignancy. Herein, we will discuss the cytopathologic findings of several solid pancreatic lesions, including acute pancreatitis, chronic pancreatitis, autoimmune pancreatitis, paraduodenal or groove pancreatitis, and other mass lesions, such as intrapancreatic accessory spleen and abscess. The key cytological features, ancillary studies, and differential diagnoses will also be discussed.

© 2020 S. Karger AG, Basel

Solid pancreatic lesions often present incidentally due to the widespread use of modern imaging techniques. They may also present with a wide range of signs and symptoms, from mild to severe, most of which are non-specific to any given entity. So-called benign lesions can present acutely when the pancreatic location influences the integrity of the ductal system. Clinical diagnoses involving the pancreas are not always straightforward, frequently calling for a comprehensive array of laboratory and radiologic testing, in the setting of appropriate clinical correlation. The use of endoscopic ultrasound-guided fine-needle aspiration (FNA) in the assessment of solid pancreatic lesions is commonly employed as a less-invasive method of definitive tissue diagnosis. Here we will cover the most significant solid, mass-forming, non-neoplastic lesions of the pancreas, including acute and chronic pancreatitis, autoimmune pancreatitis (AIP), paraduodenal or groove pancreatitis, and intrapancreatic accessory spleen (IPAS). Using the standardized nomenclature proposed by the Papanicolaou society of cytopathology, these are placed in the negative category [1].

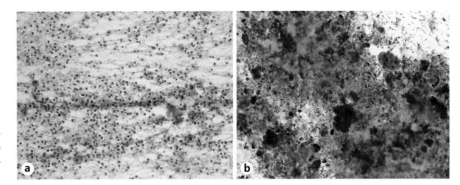

Fig. 1. Acute pancreatitis. **a** Mixed neutrophilic and histiocytic inflammation. Papanicolaou stain. **b** Background debris with calcifications. Papanicolaou stain.

The Pancreatitides

Before rendering a tissue diagnosis of any form of pancreatitis, the clinical history, laboratory findings, and imaging characteristics should be heavily weighed. A spectrum of both the clinical symptoms and tissue findings progressively correlate with the time course of episodic pancreatitis, as acute and chronic pancreatitis many times coexist within a disease spectrum.

The cytological features of chronic pancreatitis and its variants may share overlapping features, often making an accurate diagnosis difficult, without the context of the clinical and imaging findings. The key differential diagnosis for all the types of pancreatitis is the differentiation of reactive ductal atypia from adenocarcinoma. The approach to this differential diagnosis will be summarized at the end of this section.

Acute Pancreatitis

Acute pancreatitis is an acute inflammatory process of the pancreas, most often caused by gallstones and alcohol in the USA and Western countries. The revised Atlanta classification for acute pancreatitis requires that two or more of the following criteria be met for the diagnosis of acute pancreatitis: abdominal pain suggestive of pancreatitis, serum amylase, or lipase level greater than three times the upper normal value, or characteristic imaging findings [2]. The abdominal pain caused by acute pancreatitis begins in the epigastrium and may radiate to the back in approximately half of cases, may be swift in onset, is frequently unbearable, and persists without relief for 24 h. Nausea and vomiting are accompanying symptoms. The pain may lead to extreme abdominal tenderness and guarding on physical examination

[3]. Contrast-enhanced CT imaging is the preferred method for visualizing the pancreas in acute pancreatitis. General imaging findings of acute pancreatitis on CT scan include enlargement of the pancreas with diffuse edema, heterogeneity of pancreatic parenchyma, peripancreatic stranding, and peripancreatic fluid collections [3]. Pancreatitis can be further classified into interstitial edematous pancreatitis and necrotizing pancreatitis using specific CT scan imaging criteria, with the necrotizing forms carrying a worse prognosis [4]. The histology will depend on whether it is acute interstitial pancreatitis or the acute necrotizing type. The acute interstitial type is characterized by an acute inflammatory cell infiltrate, edema, and a fibrinous exudate. The acute necrotizing type is characterized by patchy necrosis, diffuse interstitial edema due to microvascular leakage, fat necrosis, neutrophils, acinar and blood vessel destruction, and interstitial hemorrhage.

Acute pancreatitis is rarely sampled by FNA. Aspirates would show neutrophilic inflammation, macrophages, debris, necrotic fat, calcium salts, and degenerating acinar and reactive ductal cells (Fig. 1a, b) [5].

Key Cytologic Features
- Dirty background with debris
- Neutrophilic inflammation
- Degenerated acinar cells
- Reactive epithelial cells
- Calcification
- Fat necrosis
- Saponification

Ancillary Studies
Microbiological studies may be indicated if an abscess or infection are suspected.

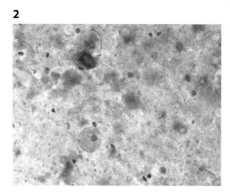
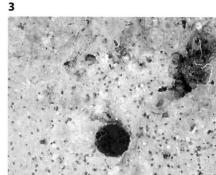

Fig. 2. Chronic pancreatitis. Dirty background, histiocytes, and calcification. Papanicolaou stain.
Fig. 3. Chronic pancreatitis. Histiocytes, giant cell with background debris and pigment. Diff-Quik stain.

Differential Diagnosis

The differential diagnosis for acute pancreatitis includes abscess and adenocarcinoma with abundant acute inflammation, due to secondary acute pancreatitis. An abscess is characterized by abundant neutrophilic inflammation. Since adenocarcinoma may be obscured by abundant acute inflammation, careful evaluation of any epithelial cells is warranted.

Chronic Pancreatitis

Chronic pancreatitis is a disease process involving progressive inflammatory changes which may cause permanent parenchymal destruction, resulting in impaired exocrine and endocrine function. Although acute pancreatitis differs temporally, both entities may coexist within a continuum. Epigastric abdominal pain with radiation to the back is the most common presenting clinical symptom. Patients may also present with malabsorptive signs of pancreatic insufficiency and diabetes.

The etiologic agents in chronic pancreatitis are nearly the same as acute pancreatitis. The majority of cases are due to alcohol abuse, ductal obstruction, and either systemic, autoimmune, or genetic disorders. Ductal obstruction is commonly due to gallstones, but can occur due to any anatomic deformity of the pancreatic parenchyma, such as tumors or cysts. Systemic diseases such as hypertriglyceridemia and systemic lupus erythematosus have also been implicated [6]. Several genetic mutations have been associated with hereditary pancreatitis. The most common mutations implicated involve the *PRSS1*, *CFTR*, *SPINK1*, and *CTRC* genes [7].

While there is no universally accepted single clinical diagnostic algorithm for chronic pancreatitis, several classification systems exist and there are broad categories of clinical testing that can be employed to support the diagnosis [8].

Serum amylase and lipase levels may be mildly elevated, but are more commonly normal due to patchy focal disease and significant parenchymal fibrosis. Serum bilirubin and alkaline phosphatase may be elevated due to ductal system compression by edema or fibrosis. Fecal elastase is the test of choice to assess for pancreatic insufficiency [9], but a 72-h quantitative fecal fat determination can also be used.

Various imaging modalities may be used due to comparable sensitivities and specificities, which include transabdominal ultrasound, CT, MRI, endoscopic retrograde cholangiopancreatography, and endoscopic ultrasound [10]. The diagnosis of chronic pancreatitis can be confirmed if calcifications are detected within the pancreas on CT scan, there is an abnormal pancreatogram with beading of the main pancreatic duct, or with an abnormal secretin pancreatic function test.

The histologic findings of affected pancreatic tissue are commensurate with the duration and severity of disease. Earlier stages will show inflammation involving the lobules, with variable destruction of acini. Inflammatory cell infiltrates, hemorrhage, and residual acinar cells will vary depending on the disease stage and progression. Calcifications will develop in chronic disease. Tissue sections show prominent parenchymal fibrosis with ductal distortion. In later stages, the pancreas may show complete loss of pancreatic acini and ducts, with only fibrosis and residual islet cells [11].

Aspirates will often show scant cellularity due to fibrosis, and minimal to mild inflammation. The background is dirty or inflammatory (Fig. 2). Inflammation is most commonly a combination of neutrophils, lymphocytes, and macrophages, often containing hemosiderin. Giant cells are usually rare (Fig. 3). Fibrotic acinar tissue may be identified (Fig. 4). Islet cells may be present but are not always seen. Metaplastic squamous cells, fat necrosis, and calcifications may also be present (Fig. 5). Granulation tissue, fibroblasts,

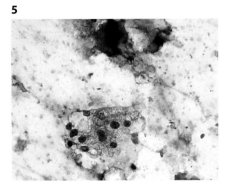

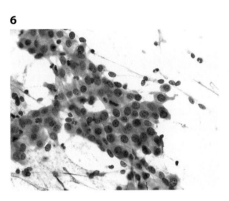

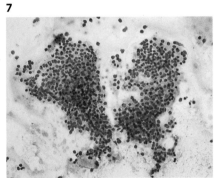

Fig. 4. Chronic pancreatitis. Acinar tissue replaced by fibrosis. Only a few residual acinar cells are attached.
Fig. 5. Chronic pancreatitis. Histiocytes and calcifications. Diff-Quik stain.

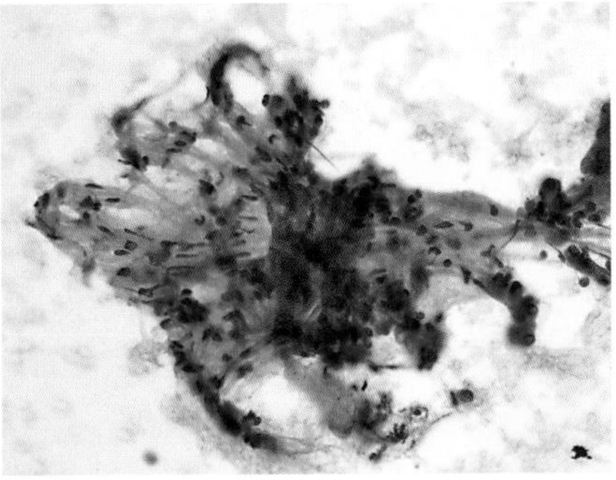

Fig. 6. Reactive ductal epithelium. A flat group of ductal cells, with nuclear enlargement. A normal mitotic figure is noted. Papanicolaou stain.
Fig. 7. Pseudohyperplastic islet cells. The islet cells are in cohesive groups. The cytoplasm is scant, and the nuclei are round to oval. When groups such as these are prominent on FNA smear, they may be mistaken for neuroendocrine tumor. Diff-Quik stain.

and reactive mesothelial cells have also been described. The residual ductal epithelium may be mildly atypical (Fig. 6) [5, 12].

In late-stage chronic pancreatitis, the pancreatic parenchyma is completely replaced by fibrosis, with only residual nests of islet cells. This pattern of pseudohyperplastic islet cells is problematic both on histopathology and cytopathology, as these groups may be mistaken for neuroendocrine tumor. Residual islet cells are cohesive (Fig. 7). The nuclei are round to oval, with smooth nuclear membranes and salt and pepper chromatin. The cytoplasm is scant and wispy.

Key Cytologic Features
- Scant cellularity
- Fibrous tissue fragments
- Mixed inflammatory cells with predominant macrophages
- Rare giant cells
- Residual islet cells
- Squamous metaplasia
- Fat necrosis
- Mild ductal epithelial atypia

Ancillary Studies
There are no ancillary studies specific to the diagnosis of chronic pancreatitis. Residual islet cells retain expression for both insulin and glucagon.

Differential Diagnosis
The pseudohyperplastic islet cells may be mistaken for a neuroendocrine tumor. Smears from a neuroendocrine tumor are hypercellular and composed of a dyshesive population of monotonous neoplastic cells, most typically with a plasmacytoid appearance. Aspirates from chronic pancreatitis will have a few cohesive groups of islet cells, with scant, wispy cytoplasm [see the chapter by Dhillon; this vol., pp. 34–41]. The differential diagnosis also includes other forms of pancreatitis.

Autoimmune Pancreatitis

AIP is a chronic fibroinflammatory disease causing diffuse pancreatic fibrosis and dysfunction, responsive to steroid therapy [13]. Two types with distinct clinicopathological features have been defined: type 1 AIP, or lymphoplasmacytic sclerosing pancreatitis, and type 2 AIP, or idiopathic

8

9

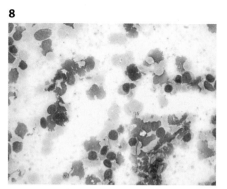
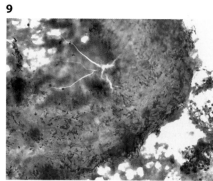

Fig. 8. AIP. The inflammatory infiltrate is a mixture of lymphocytes with plasma cells. Diff-Quik stain.

Fig. 9. AIP. Stromal fragment with a lympho-plasmacytic infiltrate and crush artifact. Diff-Quik stain.

duct-centric chronic pancreatitis. Type 1 AIP is a systemic disease, is more common, and is part of the spectrum of IgG4-related systemic disease [14]. Type 2 AIP disease is confined to the pancreas. Type 1 AIP presents with jaundice and abdominal pain, shows a male-to-female ratio of 3:1, and occurs in patients aged in their 60s. Involvement of other organs is a clue. Patients with type 2 AIP often present with acute pancreatitis. This disease affects a younger age group than type 1 AIP (median age 31 years), and there is no gender predilection [13]. Type 2 may co-occur with inflammatory bowel disease. Only type 1 AIP is associated with elevated serum levels of IgG4.

On imaging, type 1 AIP presents with diffuse parenchymal enlargement, with effacement of the lobular contour of the pancreas, giving the pancreas a "sausage shape." A halo is fairly characteristic. Type 2 AIP presents with a focal mass or diffuse pancreatic enlargement. A characteristic imaging feature of type 2 AIP is the pancreatic tail cut-off sign [14]. As both forms may present with a focal mass, the imaging differential may include pancreatic neoplasia.

The three diagnostic histopathological features of type 1 AIP are lymphoplasmacytic infiltrate, obliterative phlebitis, and storiform fibrosis. Type 2 AIP may have some of these features. Unique to type 2 AIP is the granulocyte epithelial lesions – intraluminal and intraepithelial neutrophils in medium-sized and small ducts with or without acinar inflammation, often forming neutrophilic abscesses and associated with ductal destruction and ductal ulceration [14, 15].

One study focused on the cytological criteria of AIP, and at the time of this study the two types of AIP had not been defined [16]. The features differentiating AIP from chronic pancreatitis included a relatively increased number of stromal fragments, an increased number of lymphocytes (>30 per 60× microscope objective field; Fig. 8), and cellular stromal fragments. Most cases lacked a ductal component. A few cases had ductal cells with a neutrophilic infiltrate. Frag-

ments of fibrous stromal tissue were common and usually displayed marked crush artifact (Fig. 9). The stroma was generally hypercellular, with lymphocytes and plasma cells. Cases show significantly more fragments of fibrous tissue with embedded atrophic acinar cells (Fig. 10). Based on the current classification, theoretically, the samples with a neutrophilic ductal infiltrate are consistent with type 2 AIP, and those with a prominent lymphoplasmacytic infiltrate are more consistent with type 1 AIP.

Key Cytological Features
- Numerous stromal fragments, with or without a lymphoplasmacytic infiltrate
- Lymphoplasmacytic inflammation is prominent (type 1)
- Neutrophilic infiltration of ductal cells (type 2)
- Mild atypia in ductal cells
- Absence of neutrophils, debris, and calcification in the background

Ancillary Studies
Type 1 AIP is characterized by an increase in IgG4-positive plasma cells. The recommended number is >10/HPF when assessing a core biopsy. The IgG4/IgG ratio is not as helpful [17].

Differential Diagnosis
The differential diagnosis includes other types of chronic pancreatitis. Adenocarcinoma is in the differential diagnosis of reactive ductal atypia.

Paraduodenal/Groove Pancreatitis

Groove pancreatitis is an uncommon form of focal chronic pancreatitis, which affects the space or "groove" adjacent to the duodenum, pancreatic head, and common bile duct.

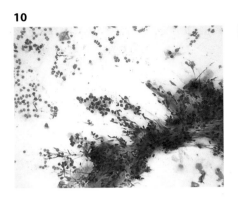
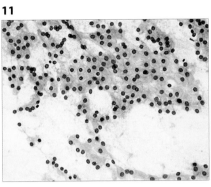

Fig. 10. AIP. Stromal fragment with attached acinar cells and lymphocytic infiltrate with crush artifact. Diff-Quik stain.

Fig. 11. Groove pancreatitis. Bland, mucinous epithelium from Brunner's glands. Papanicolaou stain. Photo courtesy of Dr. Edward Stelow, Department of Pathology, University of Virginia.

Groove pancreatitis is often misdiagnosed as pancreatic malignancy or AIP due to the clinical signs and symptoms in conjunction with radiologic findings, including pseudotumor formation [18]. Imaging techniques such as transabdominal ultrasonography typically show thickening of the duodenal wall, suprapapillar luminal stenosis, a hypoechoic mass within the groove area between the duodenum and pancreatic head, with cysts and an irregular duodenal surface. The common bile duct may show mild to moderate dilatation.

Cytological samples share many of the traits seen in chronic pancreatitis, as well as the presence of bland mucinous glands (Brunner's glands; Fig. 11), with the stromal component very cellular and spindled, often mimicking mesenchymal neoplasia. The stromal fragments are usually moderately cellular and may have admixed lymphocytes [19].

Key Cytological Features
- Fragments of cellular stroma, occasionally with inflammation
- Bland Brunner's gland epithelium
- Mildly atypical ductal epithelium

Ancillary Studies
The spindled stromal cells may show immunoreactivity with antibodies to smooth muscle actin (SMA) [19].

Differential Diagnosis of All the Pancreatitides
The differential diagnosis and challenges on FNA will include differentiating among the various types of pancreatitis and differentiating reactive ductal atypia from adenocarcinoma.

Recognizing AIP
Recognition of specific forms of pancreatitis require correlation with clinical and imaging findings. Each type is sum-

marized in Table 1. In chronic pancreatitis, unlike AIP, tissue fragments do not usually contain clusters of lymphocytes and plasma cells, although scattered lymphocytes, plasma cells, macrophages, and siderophages are often seen sparsely associated with background fibrotic fragments. Debris consistent with intraductal secretions, as well as calcifications, are typically seen in chronic pancreatitis, but not AIP. Ancillary studies for IgG4 will be helpful to diagnose type 1 AIP.

Reactive Atypia versus Adenocarcinoma
The cytological atypia accompanying inflammatory processes may be difficult to differentiate from adenocarcinoma (Fig. 12), and adenocarcinoma may be associated with cytological findings of pancreatitis. Features that differentiate adenocarcinoma from reactive atypia include alterations in the architecture of the groups, with overlapping and crowding of the nuclei. In carcinoma, the cells are enlarged greater than 1.5 times the size of a red blood cell on air-dried smears, show abnormalities of chromatin distribution, and irregularities of chromatin distribution, being either hyperchromatic or hypochromatic. Single malignant cells and groups with anisonucleosis of greater than 4:1 are diagnostic. Any atypical mitotic figure is also diagnostic, although normal mitoses may be encountered in reactive processes. The cytomorphological features of ductal adenocarcinoma are reviewed in detail in the chapter by Dhillon [this vol., pp. 74–91].

Ancillary studies for the differential diagnosis of reactive ductal atypia from adenocarcinoma have been recently reviewed [20]. A number of proteins have been identified that are overexpressed in pancreatic ductal adenocarcinoma (PDAC) compared to benign/reactive ductal epithelium. These include maspin, S100 calcium binding protein P (S100P), U3 small nucleolar ribonucleoprotein (IMP3), CK17, and mesothelin. The tumor-suppressor genes

Table 1. Clinicopathologic features and cytopathology of various forms of pancreatitis

Disease	Etiology	Age	Gender	Laboratory features	Imaging	Cytological features
Acute pancreatitis	Alcohol Gallstones Trauma Others	Adults, no age predilection	Alcohol related: M>F Gallstone related: M<F	Elevated serum amylase and lipase	Depends on the severity of disease Diffuse enlargement, edema, peripancreatic fluid collections Necrosis in severe cases	Background debris and saponification Fat necrosis Variable neutrophilic inflammation Epithelial atypia
Chronic pancreatitis, NOS	Alcohol Gallstones Hereditary syndromes	5th decade and older	M>F	Pancreatic insufficiency	Pancreatic duct tapering and beading Calcifications	Background debris, calcifications Inflammation variable Loss of acinar component Stromal fragments and few residual ductal groups Islet cells occasionally prominent
Type 1AIP (LPSP)	IgG4 related	6th to 7th decade	M>F	Elevated serum IgG4	Diffusely enlarged or mass lesion Halo	Stromal fragments numerous, usually cellular with lymphocytes and plasma cells, or crush artifact Stromal fragments with acinar cells and lymphoplasmacytic inflammation Mild ductal atypia
Type 2 AIP (IDCP)	Unknown	4th and 5th decades	M = F	None	Mass lesion or diffuse enlargement Pancreatic tail cut-off sign	Stromal fragments numerous Ductal groups with neutrophilic inflammation Mild ductal atypia
Groove/ paraduodenal pancreatitis	Alcohol Other anatomic contributing factors	5th or 6th decade	M>F	None	Soft tissue mass, with or without cysts Location: paraduodenal groove	Bland, mucinous glands Numerous stromal fragments

CDKN2a (encoding p16 protein), *TP53*, and mothers against decapentaplegic homolog 4 (*SMAD4/DPC4*) are either deleted or mutated in PDAC, and immunohistochemistry for these markers serves as a surrogate marker for malignancy. Mutations in *CDKN2A* (p16) and *DPC4* lead to a loss of the corresponding protein expression. Mutations in *TP53* lead to overexpression of the protein, p53, unless the mutation is truncating, in which case there is complete loss of expression. PDAC loses expression for von Hippel-Lindau tumor suppressor protein (pVHL). A pitfall is that S100P and maspin may both be expressed by gastric foveolar epithelium. True positive S100P staining is nuclear and cytoplasmic (Fig. 13). Since false positive and negative staining may occur with any individual antibody, it is suggested that a panel be used. DPC4 is the most specific [21]. Table 2 summarizes the ancillary studies most useful for this differential diagnosis.

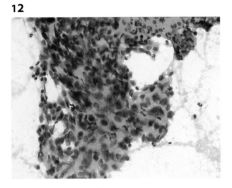

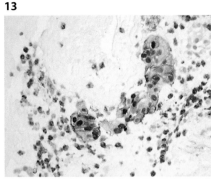

Fig. 12. Severe atypia. This sheet shows crowded, overlapping nuclei that are enlarged, with hyperchromasia. There is neutrophilic inflammation. The differential diagnosis includes severe reactive atypia versus adenocarcinoma. Papanicolaou stain.

Fig. 13. S100P. True positive staining is nuclear and cytoplasmic. Cell block, immunoperoxidase stain.

Table 2. Ancillary studies for the diagnosis of adenocarcinoma [32]

Antibody	Staining pattern in PDAC	Comment
DPC4	Loss of nuclear expression in 50–60%	
p53	Nuclear expression in 60%	
CK17	Strong, cytoplasmic	
S100P	Strong nuclear and cytoplasmic	Nuclear and cytoplasmic expression in foveolar epithelium
		May have high background staining, improved when processed in a microwave
		Cytoplasmic in reactive ducts
IMP3	Cytoplasmic	Weaker and focal cytoplasmic expression
		False negative in small samples
Maspin	Nuclear or nuclear and cytoplasmic	Cytoplasmic expression in gastric and duodenal epithelium
pVHL	Loss of expression	Retained in normal tissues

Intrapancreatic Spleen

An accessory spleen is defined as splenic tissue in an ectopic site due to a congenital abnormality and is most often found near the splenic hilum [22]. Less commonly, they are located within the pancreatic tail, an entity known as intrapancreatic spleen (IPAS) (also termed splenule and splenunculus). IPAS can present in both asymptomatic and symptomatic individuals displaying abdominal pain and are usually incidental findings on imaging with no apparent age or sex predilection. In many instances, IPAS may mimic malignancy radiologically, with non-functioning pancreatic neuroendocrine tumor high on the list of differential diagnoses, and hypervascular focal metastasis much lower [22]. Similarly, autotransplanted splenic tissue within the abdomen, known as splenosis, has been described due to trauma or iatrogenic rupture and can mimic lymphoma or carcinoma. Proper identification can prevent unnecessary surgical procedures.

IPAS should be considered when a hypervascular mass is present within the pancreatic tail, close to the splenic hilum. This location and similar attenuation to the spleen on non-contrast and postcontrast CT at different phases is support-

ive of the diagnosis. Technetium-99m (^{99m}Tc)-labeled HDRBC scintigraphy or superparamagnetic iron oxide-enhanced MRI techniques can also be used to confirm the diagnosis of IPAS as long as certain caveats are kept in mind [22]. Unfortunately, IPAS may sometimes mildly react with octreotide scintigraphy, owing to somatostatin receptors on lymphocytes [23–25], which may additionally lead to a false positive interpretation for a neuroendocrine tumor.

Splenic white pulp consists of lymphocytes and macrophages arranged around arteries. The red pulp consists of prominent vascular sinuses, with specialized endothelial cells. The overall histology is compatible with vascularized lymphoid tissue.

Aspirates show polymorphous small lymphocytes with other inflammatory cells such as plasma cells, macrophages, neutrophils, and eosinophils. There is usually a prominent vascular component, with tangles of small capillary-like vessels, spindled cells, and associated sinus histiocytes (Fig. 14a, b) [26]. Platelet clumps are also sometimes seen (Fig. 15) [27]. At first glance, findings recapitulate a benign lymph node; however, IPAS tissue will usually be devoid of tingible-body macrophages and germinal center aggregates.

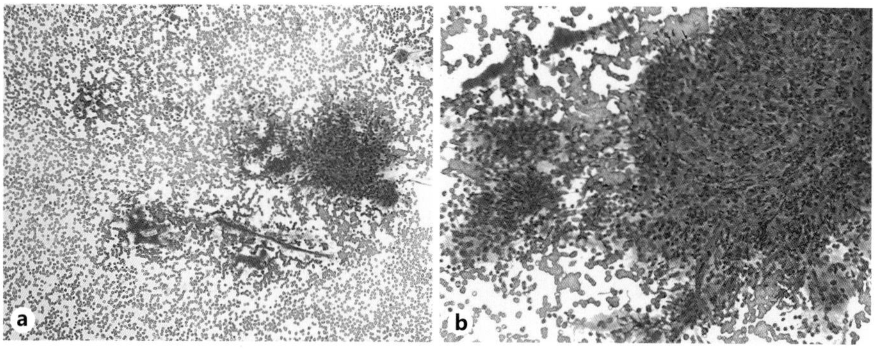

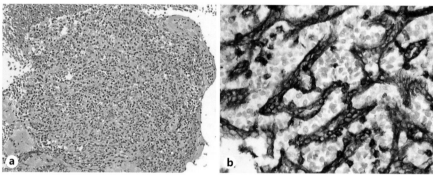

Fig. 14. Intrapancreatic spleen. **a** Low-power view showing an aggregate of lymphocytes with a central arteriole, and numerous background lymphocytes. Diff-Quik stain. **b** Numerous lymphocytes and histiocytes attached to an arteriole. Diff-Quik stain.

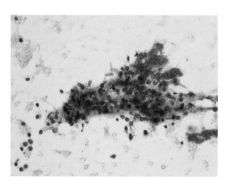

Fig. 15. Intrapancreatic spleen. Lymphocytes and platelet aggregates. Papanicolaou stain.

Fig. 16. Intrapancreatic spleen. **a** Cell block with cohesive fragments showing small vessels. HE stain. **b** The capillaries are identified with CD8. Cell block, immunoperoxidase stain.

Key Cytological Features
- Mixed population of lymphocytes
- Prominent vascular component, with tangles of small capillary-like vessels, spindled cells, and associated sinus histiocytes
- Platelet aggregates
- Absent epithelial cells unless there is a contaminant
- Absent tingible body macrophages and germinal centers

Ancillary Studies
CD8 and CD31 immunohistochemical staining within the splenic sinus endothelial cells is confirmatory (Fig. 16a, b) [26].

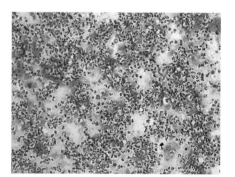

Fig. 17. Pancreatic abscess. Abundant neutrophils. Diff-Quik stain.

Differential Diagnosis
The differential diagnosis includes pancreatic neuroendocrine tumors because of the imaging findings, benign lymph node tissue, and lymphoma. CD8 immunostaining highlights splenic sinusoidal endothelium. A CD45 immunostain performed alongside neuroendocrine markers can discriminate between cells of hematopoietic origin versus a neuroendocrine neoplasm and/or normal islet cell aggregates. If there is concern for a hematopoietic malignancy, immunophenotyping is recommended through either immunohistochemistry or flow cytometry.

Pancreatic Abscess

Pancreatic abscess (PA) formation is commonly seen as a complication of acute pancreatitis and/or pseudocyst infection, although several reports of PA due to other causes exist, such as secondary infection [28, 29], penetrating duodenal ulcer, and pancreas divisum. PAs are defined as well-circumscribed collections of pus within the pancreas, without significant pancreatic necrosis. Management usually involves the administration of antibiotic therapy in conjunction with endoscopic ultrasound-guided drainage and debridement, with an occasional requirement for stent placement [30].

PAs can manifest clinically severe signs and symptoms highly suspicious for malignancy such as abdominal pain, fever, weight loss, and obstructive jaundice. CA19-9 levels can become elevated and imaging may show low-density parenchymal areas within the pancreas and adjacent liver parenchyma [31].

The histology of a PA is the same as that of an abscess from any location. Histology will depict an admixture of neutrophilic and necrotic fibrinous debris gathered from a localized collection. Giant cells and lymphocytes may also be present. The cytological samples will show abundant acute inflammation, necrotic debris, and histiocytes (Fig. 17).

Key Cytological Features
- Neutrophils
- Lymphocytes and giant cells may also be present
- Necrotic debris
- Predominantly an absence of epithelial element

Ancillary Testing
Ancillary studies will focus on identifying microbial organisms.

Differential Diagnosis
Although abscesses usually produce straightforward cytologic findings, tumor diatheses from an associated malignancy can appear similar. Furthermore, an abscess may coexist with a hidden component of adenocarcinoma.

Disclosure Statement

The authors have nothing to disclose.

References

1 Pitman MB, Centeno BA, Ali SZ, Genevay M, Stelow E, Mino-Kenudson M, Castillo CF, Schmidt CM, Brugge WR, Layfield LJ: Standardized terminology and nomenclature for pancreatobiliary cytology: The Papanicolaou Society of Cytopathology Guidelines. Cytojournal 2014; 11(suppl 1):3.
2 Quinlan JD: Acute pancreatitis. Am Fam Physician 2014;90:632–639.
3 Banks PA, Freeman ML; Practice Parameters Committee of the American College of Gastroenterology: Practice guidelines in acute pancreatitis. Am J Gastroenterol 2006;101:2379–2400.
4 Foster BR, Jensen KK, Bakis G, Shaaban AM, Coakley FV: Revised Atlanta Classification for Acute Pancreatitis: a pictorial essay. Radiographics 2016;36:675–687.
5 Conrad R, Castelino-Prabhu S, Cobb C, Raza A: Cytopathology of the pancreatobiliary tract – the agony, and sometimes, the ease of it. J Gastrointest Oncol 2013;4:210–219.
6 Pham A, Forsmark C: Chronic pancreatitis: review and update of etiology, risk factors, and management. F1000Res 2018;7:607.
7 Raphael KL, Willingham FF: Hereditary pancreatitis: current perspectives. Clin Exp Gastroenterol 2016;9:197–207.
8 Duggan SN, Ni Chonchubhair HM, Lawal O, O'Connor DB, Conlon KC: Chronic pancreatitis: a diagnostic dilemma. World J Gastroenterol 2016; 22:2304–2313.
9 Lee LS, Tabak YP, Kadiyala V, Sun X, Suleiman S, Johannes RS, Banks PA, Conwell DL: Diagnosis of chronic pancreatitis incorporating endosonographic features, demographics, and behavioral risk. Pancreas 2017;46:405–409.
10 Issa Y, Kempeneers MA, van Santvoort HC, Bollen TL, Bipat S, Boermeester MA: Diagnostic performance of imaging modalities in chronic pancreatitis: a systematic review and meta-analysis. Eur Radiol 2017;27:3820–3844.
11 Kloppel G, Adsay NV: Chronic pancreatitis and the differential diagnosis versus pancreatic cancer. Arch Pathol Lab Med 2009;133:382–387.
12 Stelow EB, Bardales RH, Lai R, Mallery S, Linzie BM, Crary GS, Stanley MW: The cytological spectrum of chronic pancreatitis. Diagn Cytopathol 2005;32:65–69.
13 Majumder S, Takahashi N, Chari ST: Autoimmune pancreatitis. Dig Dis Sci 2017;62:1762–1769.
14 Deshpande V, Gupta R, Sainani N, Sahani DV, Virk R, Ferrone C, Khosroshahi A, Stone JH, Lauwers GY: Subclassification of autoimmune pancreatitis: a histologic classification with clinical significance. Am J Surg Pathol 2011;35:26–35.
15 Notohara K, Burgart LJ, Yadav D, Chari S, Smyrk TC: Idiopathic chronic pancreatitis with periductal lymphoplasmacytic infiltration: clinicopathologic features of 35 cases. Am J Surg Pathol 2003; 27:1119–1127.
16 Deshpande V, Mino-Kenudson M, Brugge WR, Pitman MB, Fernandez-del Castillo C, Warshaw AL, Lauwers GY: Endoscopic ultrasound guided fine needle aspiration biopsy of autoimmune pancreatitis: diagnostic criteria and pitfalls. Am J Surg Pathol 2005;29:1464–1471.
17 Deshpande V, Zen Y, Chan JK, Yi EE, Sato Y, Yoshino T, et al: Consensus statement on the pathology of IgG4-related disease. Mod Pathol 2012;25: 1181–1192.

18 Levenick JM, Gordon SR, Sutton JE, Suriawinata A, Gardner TB: A comprehensive, case-based review of groove pancreatitis. Pancreas 2009; 38:e169–e175.

19 Chute DJ, Stelow EB: Fine-needle aspiration features of paraduodenal pancreatitis (groove pancreatitis): a report of three cases. Diagn Cytopathol 2012;40:1116–1121.

20 Misdraji J, Centeno BA, Pitman MB: Ancillary tests in the diagnosis of liver and pancreatic neoplasms. Cancer Cytopathol 2018;126(suppl 8): 672–690.

21 Sweeney J, Rao R, Margolskee E, Goyal A, Heymann JJ, Siddiqui MT: Immunohistochemical staining for S100P, SMAD4, and IMP3 on cell block preparations is sensitive and highly specific for pancreatic ductal adenocarcinoma. J Am Soc Cytopathol 2018;7:318–323.

22 Kawamoto S, Johnson PT, Hall H, Cameron JL, Hruban RH, Fishman EK: Intrapancreatic accessory spleen: CT appearance and differential diagnosis. Abdom Imaging 2012;37:812–827.

23 Bhutiani N, Egger ME, Doughtie CA, Burkardt ES, Scoggins CR, Martin RC, 2nd, McMasters KM: Intrapancreatic accessory spleen (IPAS): a single-institution experience and review of the literature. Am J Surg 2017;213:816–820.

24 Suriano S, Ceriani L, Gertsch P, Crippa S, Giovanella L: Accessory spleen mimicking a pancreatic neuroendocrine tumor. Tumori 2011;97: 39e–41e.

25 Brasca LE, Zanello A, De Gaspari A, De Cobelli F, Zerbi A, Fazio F, Del Maschio A: Intrapancreatic accessory spleen mimicking a neuroendocrine tumor: magnetic resonance findings and possible diagnostic role of different nuclear medicine tests. Eur Radiol 2004;14:1322–1323.

26 Schreiner AM, Mansoor A, Faigel DO, Morgan TK: Intrapancreatic accessory spleen: mimic of pancreatic endocrine tumor diagnosed by endoscopic ultrasound-guided fine-needle aspiration biopsy. Diagn Cytopathol 2008;36:262–265.

27 Conway AB, Cook SM, Samad A, Attam R, Pambuccian SE: Large platelet aggregates in endoscopic ultrasound-guided fine-needle aspiration of the pancreas and peripancreatic region: a clue for the diagnosis of intrapancreatic or accessory spleen. Diagn Cytopathol 2013;41:661–672.

28 Liu Q, He Z, Bie P: Solitary pancreatic tuberculous abscess mimicking prancreatic cystadenocarcinoma: a case report. BMC Gastroenterol 2003;3:1.

29 Kumar S, Bandyopadhyay MK, Bhattacharyya K, Ghosh T, Bandyopadhyay M, Ghosh RR: A rare case of pancreatic abscess due to candida tropicalis. J Glob Infect Dis 2011;3:396–398.

30 Ge N, Liu X, Wang S, Wang G, Guo J, Liu W, Sun S: Treatment of pancreatic abscess with endoscopic ultrasound-guided placement of a covered metal stent following failed balloon dilation and endoscopic necrosectomy. Endosc Ultrasound 2012;1: 110–113.

31 Shulik O, Cavanagh Y, Grossman M: Pancreatic lesion: malignancy or abscess? Am J Case Rep 2016;17:337–339.

32 Liu H, Shi J, Anandan V, Wang HL, Diehl D, Blansfield J, Gerhard G, Lin F: Reevaluation and identification of the best immunohistochemical panel (pVHL, maspin, S100P, IMP-3) for ductal adenocarcinoma of the pancreas. Arch Pathol Lab Med 2012;136:601–609.

Prof. Barbara A. Centeno
Department of Pathology, Moffitt Cancer Center
12902 USF Magnolia Drive
Tampa, FL 33612 (USA)
barbara.centeno@moffitt.org

Chapter 6

Published online: September 29, 2020

Centeno BA, Dhillon J (eds): Pancreatic Tumors. Monogr Clin Cytol. Basel, Karger, 2020, vol 26, pp 53–73 (DOI:10.1159/000455735)

Non-Neoplastic and Neoplastic Cysts of the Pancreas

Barbara A. Centeno[a, b]   Sarah C. Thomas[c]

[a]Department of Pathology, Moffitt Cancer Center, Tampa, FL, USA; [b]Department of Oncologic Sciences, Morsani College of Medicine, University of South Florida, Tampa, FL, USA; [c]Office of Chief Medical Examiner, New York, NY, USA

Abstract

Inflammatory, developmental, and neoplastic lesions may all present as cystic masses on imaging. Pseudocyst is the most common of these and presents in association with a history of pancreatitis. Pancreatic cystic neoplasms are uncommon compared to solid neoplasms. They often present incidentally; therefore, an incidentally discovered cyst in the pancreas should be assessed with a high index of suspicion for neoplasm. The most common and frequently encountered cystic neoplasms include serous cystadenoma, mucinous cystic neoplasm, and intraductal papillary mucinous neoplasm. Less common epithelial cystic neoplasms include acinar cell cystadenoma and cystadenocarcinoma. Any solid neoplasm occurring in the pancreas or vicinity of the pancreas that has undergone cystic degeneration may present as a cystic mass. Non-epithelial lesions, such as lymphangioma, are also included in the differential diagnosis. The work-up needs to begin with a review of the clinical and imaging findings to establish a differential diagnosis. The primary focus of the pathologist will be first on differentiating mucinous from non-mucinous entities, since this will determine if the mass is an intraductal papillary mucinous neoplasm or a mucinous cystic neoplasm. If it is mucinous, the next step is to determine if the cystic neoplasm contains cells with high-grade cytological features. If it is non-mucinous, the pathologist needs to assess for neoplastic cells that would indicate a different neoplastic process. The cytological features need to be integrated with cyst fluid carcinoembryonic antigen and amylase measurements. Currently, molecular pathology is being integrated into the analysis of pancreatic cyst fluids. Here we will cover the cytological features and ancillary findings in cystic masses of the pancreas.

© 2020 S. Karger AG, Basel

Pancreatic cysts are less common than solid pancreatic masses, and include inflammatory, developmental, and neoplastic cysts (Table 1). The majority are pancreatic pseudocysts. Serous cystadenoma (SCA), intraductal papillary mucinous neoplasm (IPMN), and mucinous cystic neoplasm (MCN) are the most common cystic neoplasms [1, 2]. IPMN and MCN are precursors for the development of pancreatic ductal adenocarcinoma (PDAC). Many cystic neoplasms are identified incidentally during imaging for an unrelated reason, and the majority of incidentally discovered cysts are IPMN and, less commonly, MCN [3]. The purpose of pancreatic cyst fluid (PCF) analysis is to differentiate non-neoplastic from neoplastic cysts, particularly mucinous cysts, and to identify the risk of malignancy, in order to determine the correct management.

Table 1. Cystic lesions

Non-neoplastic	Neoplastic
Inflammatory	Primarily cystic
Pseudocyst	Acinar cell cystadenocarcinoma
Infections	Mucinous cystic neoplasm
Abscesses	Serous cystadenoma
Hydatid cyst	Primarily intraductal neoplasms
Cysticercosis	Intraductal papillary mucinous neoplasm
Tuberculosis	Intraductal papillary oncocytic neoplasm
Epithelial cysts – squamous lining	Intraductal tubular neoplasm
Lymphoepithelial cyst	Solid neoplasms with cystic degeneration
Epidermoid cyst in intrapancreatic spleen	Neuroendocrine tumor
Squamoid cyst	Solid pseudopapillary neoplasm
Epithelial cysts – other epithelial lining	Mesenchymal neoplasms
Acinar cystic transformation	Schwannoma
Von Hippel-Lindau	Gastrointestinal stromal tumor
Adult polycystic kidney disease	Hemangioma
Cystic fibrosis	Lymphangioma
Rare cystic lesions	
Cystic hamartoma	
Congenital cysts	
Endometriotic cyst	
Enteric cysts/ciliated cyst	
Retention cyst	

Multimodal Approach to Pancreatic Cyst Diagnosis

The approach to the diagnosis of pancreatic cysts needs to be multimodal, incorporating clinical and imaging findings with the cytological findings and ancillary test results.

Clinical
Many pancreatic cystic masses are discovered incidentally. Symptoms, when present, relate to the presence of an abdominal mass, and include abdominal pain, nausea, and vomiting. Age and gender distributions have been described for the various pancreatic cysts. For example, MCN is known to occur predominantly in females in the sixth and seventh decades of life. Solid pseudopapillary neoplasm (SPN) has a strong female predilection and occurs mostly in younger patients.

Imaging
The imaging pattern is essential to formulating a preoperative differential diagnosis. Sureka et al. [4] summarized the various imaging patterns of cystic lesions of the pancreas which can be used to formulate a differential diagnosis (Fig. 1). The patterns include: unilocular, microcystic with a central scar, macrocystic, cystic with a solid component,

macrocystic with calcifications, and cyst with ductal communication. The differential diagnosis of various imaging presentations is summarized in Table 2. The enhancement pattern also contributes to the cyst classification. Some are associated with calcifications. The macrocystic pattern with peripheral calcifications is typical of MCN and may occur with lymphoepithelial cyst of the pancreas (LECP). Septal calcifications are a feature of branch duct (BD)-IPMN, LECP, and lymphangioma, and pseudocyst may be associated with rim calcifications [4].

Cytological Evaluation
Cytological assessment begins with the evaluation of the gross appearance of the PCF. The next step is to evaluate the slides at low power to assess the background, cellularity, and cellular composition of the smears. The architectural features of any groups may be evident at low power, including the degree of cellular cohesion. At high power, the detailed nuclear and cytoplasmic features are assessed.

Ancillary Testing
Ancillary studies are crucial for differentiating mucinous from non-mucinous lesions, and for identifying lesions at risk of harboring malignancy, as often the cyst fluid lacks

Table 2. Differential diagnosis of pancreatic cysts according to imaging patterns [3]

Unilocular	Micro-cystic	Macro-cystic	Cystic transformation of pancreas	Cyst with ductal communication	Multi-focal	Solid-cystic
Pseudocyst	SCA	MCN	Dysontogenetic cyst	IPMN	BD-IPMN	SPN
Cystic PanNET		BD-IPMN	Cystic fibrosis	Retention cysts	Pseudo-cysts	Pancreatoblastoma
MCN		Lymphangioma	Disseminated SCA	Post-pancreatitis collections	SCA	Cystic degeneration in solid tumors
Unilocular SCA		LECP	Congenital syndromes			Malignant transformation of cystic neoplasm
Retention cyst		Infectious cyst				Hemorrhagic pseudocyst
Developmental cyst		Duplication cyst				
Epithelial cyst		Mesothelial cyst				
Epidermoid cyst in intrapancreatic spleen		Oligocystic SCA				
Infectious cyst						
Endometrial cyst						

MCN, mucinous cystic neoplasm; PanNET, pancreatic neuroendocrine tumor; SCA, serous cystadenoma; LECP, lymphoepithelial cyst; IPMN, intraductal papillary mucinous neoplasm; BD, branch duct; MD, main duct; SPN, solid pseudopapillary neoplasm.

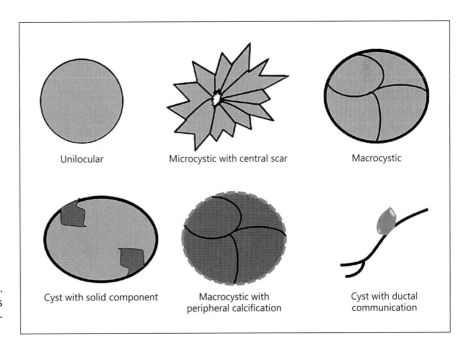

Fig. 1. Reproduced from Sureka et al. [4]. Figure 1. Line diagram illustrating various morphology of cystic pancreatic lesions. Licensed under CC-BY.

Unilocular

Microcystic with central scar

Macrocystic

Cyst with solid component

Macrocystic with peripheral calcification

Cyst with ductal communication

neoplastic cells. Ancillary studies include biochemical analysis, immunohistochemistry, and molecular analysis.

Biochemical Analysis

Current practice is to measure the PCF for carcinoembryonic antigen (CEA) and amylase levels. An elevated CEA is indicative of a mucinous cyst. A multi-institutional study established a cut-off of 192 ng/mL as the most sensitive and specific for the diagnosis of a mucinous cyst [5]. Since then, there have been a number of studies evaluating the best cut-off level, with the best cyst fluid CEA levels ranging from 48.6 to 800 ng/mL [6–9]. As the CEA level is increased, the sensitivity is decreased. Of note, a low level of CEA does not exclude a mucinous cyst, as occasionally these may have very low CEA measurements, as low as 1.6 ng/mL [10]. It is recommended that each laboratory establish its own cut-off level [11].

Cyst fluid amylase levels are very useful for excluding pseudocysts from other cyst types. An amylase level of <250 U/L has a very high specificity for excluding pseudocysts [6]. Elevated PCF levels of amylase cannot be used to differentiate IPMN from MCN [12].

Das-1 is a monoclonal antibody reactive to premalignant conditions of the gastrointestinal tract [13]. It showed a sensitivity of 85% and a specificity of 95% in tissues for detecting high-grade dysplasia and carcinoma. In PCF, it showed a sensitivity and specificity of 89 and 100%, respectively. In a cross-validation study of 169 patient PCF samples, Das-1 identified high-risk pancreatic cysts with 88% sensitivity and 99% specificity, and 95% accuracy, at a cut-off optical density value of 0.104. High-risk cysts were defined as those with invasive carcinomas, high-grade dysplasia, or intestinal-type IPMNs with intermediate-grade dysplasia [14]. This biomarker improves upon the detection of high-risk cysts and may be used in addition to other markers.

Immunohistochemistry

Immunohistochemistry is needed for the diagnosis of solid masses presenting with cystic degeneration, specifically pancreatic neuroendocrine tumor (PanNET) and solid pseudopapillary neoplasm (SPN), the diagnosis of SCA, and the diagnosis of PDAC in cysts with suspected invasion. Specifically, immunohistochemical evaluation for the protein of SMAD4/DPC4 serves as a surrogate marker of mutations in the gene. Loss of SMAD4/DPC4 expression can be used to confirm the presence of invasive carcinoma. Other markers used to confirm invasion include S100P, maspin, p53, and IMP3 [15].

Molecular

Whole-exome sequencing identified mutational profiles specific for cystic neoplasms [16]. SCAs contain a mutation in the von Hippel-Lindau (*VHL*) gene. SPNs have a single mutation in *CTNBB1*. *KRAS* and *RNF43* mutations occur in both IPMN and MCN. *GNAS* mutations are only encountered in IPMN [17, 18]. These mutations are found in PCF, and *KRAS* and *GNAS* mutations in PCF classify a cyst as a neoplastic mucinous cyst [18].

There have been a number of other studies evaluating molecular markers for the diagnosis and risk stratification of pancreatic cysts [19–22]. Alterations in *TP53*, *PIK3CA*, *PTEN*, *NOTCH1*, *SMAD* family members, and *CDKN2A* are associated with high-grade dysplasia/adenocarcinoma in pancreatic cysts. Published studies to date show that the addition of molecular testing improves the diagnosis of pancreatic cysts. A prospective study of PCF DNA testing using next-generation sequencing (NGS) showed that preoperative NGS testing of PCF for *KRAS/GNAS* and alterations in *TP53/PIK3CA/PTEN* had a sensitivity of 89% and specificity of 100% for advanced neoplasia [23]. In a multicenter trial of 130 patients, molecular analysis of PCF accurately identified the cyst type, and identified the presence of high-grade dysplasia and adenocarcinoma [24]. Molecular markers diagnostic of high-grade dysplasia or invasive carcinoma in this study were mutations in *SMAD4/DPC4*, *TP53*, LOH chromosome 17, and aneuploidy in chromosomes 5p, 8p, 13q, and 18q [24]. Table 3 summarizes the age and gender distribution, imaging, and cytological and ancillary test findings of the most common pancreatic cysts.

Non-Neoplastic Cysts

Ductal Retention Cyst

Retention cysts are a cystic dilation in the pancreatic duct incited by duct obstruction [4]. They may be congenital or secondary to obstructions caused by calculi, mucin, chronic pancreatitis, or pancreatic adenocarcinoma, and occur in cystic fibrosis [25]. The mucosal lining is cuboidal [26], or may be squamous metaplastic, denuded, or mucinous if the epithelium has been replaced by pancreatic intraepithelial neoplasia. Most are asymptomatic and merely incidental findings. They were thought to be small (3–5 mm) but have been reported as being >4 cm [26]. They are well defined, unilocular, and without mural nodules. However, their im-

Table 3. Key clinical, imaging, cytological, biochemical, and molecular findings of pancreatic cysts

Diagnosis	Age (years) and gender distribution	Imaging features	Cytology	Biochemical analysis		Molecular
				CEA	amylase	
Pseudocyst	Secondary to pancreatitis, age and gender depend on the etiology; middle aged and older males when the etiology is alcohol-induced pancreatitis	Rounded, unilocular mass Thick wall Non-septated Hypoechoic or anechoic No enhancement Rim calcifications variably present	Macrophages Yellow hematoidin-like pigment Background debris	Low	High	None
LECP	Older adults, mean age 56 years; male-to-female ratio of 4:1	Unilocular or multilocular May be peripancreatic and protrude from the pancreatic surface Thick walls, internal debris, may appear solid	Anucleated and nucleated squamous cells Cystic debris Cholesterol crystals	High	High	None
SCA	Age range 26–91 years, mean age 60 years; slight female predominance	Well-circumscribed Classic: multilocular, small cysts, central stellate scar Thin wall with septal enhancement Others: macrocystic or solid pattern (often confused with PanNET)	Scant, clear fluid Cuboidal cells in flat sheets Stripped nuclei Clear cytoplasm, or microvacuoles	Low	Low	VHL
MCN	Age range 14–95 years, mean age 40–50 years; mostly women, female-to-male ratio is 20:1	Unilocular or multilocular, septated Peripheral calcifications variable Lacks connection to pancreatic ductal system Usually in body or tail Thick septa, lacks peripheral enhancement	Background mucin Neoplastic glandular epithelium with either low-grade or high-grade epithelial atypia	High	Low or high	KRAS RNF43
IPMN	Age range 30–94 years, mean age 66 years; slightly more frequently in males than females	Connect to the ductal system MD-IPMN: dilated MPD, with or without papillae No enhancement BD-IPMN: multicystic, grape-like clusters Thin, peripheral enhancement variably present	Background mucin Neoplastic glandular epithelium with either low-grade or high-grade epithelial atypia	High	Low or high	KRAS GNAS RNF43
IOPN	Age range 20–80 years, mean age 61.6 years; male-to-female ratio 1.65:1	Complex, cystic mass, may appear solid	Oncocytic neoplastic cells Positive with MUC6	Not established	Not established	ARHGAP26 ASXL1 EPHA8 ERBB4

Table 3 (continued)

Diagnosis	Age (years) and gender distribution	Imaging features	Cytology	Biochemical analysis		Molecular
				CEA	amylase	
SPN	Most often in adolescent or young adult females (90% of all patients), range 7–79 years, mean age 28 years; in males, 25–72 years (mean 35)	Sharply demarcated, solid and cystic Calcifications uncommon Hemangioma-like progressive enhancement	Vascular cores with a central capillary and myxoid stroma Monomorphic neoplastic cells with round to oval nuclei with nuclear grooves, small nucleoli Cytoplasm variable: vacuoles, cytoplasmic tails, inclusions	Not established	Not established	CTNNB1
Cystic PanNET	Any age (30–60 years), mean age 50 years; M = F	Unilocular Thick, peripheral, solid cystic enhancement Calcifications variably present	Variably cellular Monotonous cell population High N:C ratio Round, uniform nuclei Salt and pepper chromatin Positive for neuroendocrine markers	Low	Low	None
Lymphangio-ma	All ages (mean 29 years)	Solitary, multicystic, anechoic or hypoechoic Thin septations	No mucin Mixed population of lymphocytes No epithelial cells	Low	Mildly elevated	None

MCN, mucinous cystic neoplasm; PanNET, pancreatic neuroendocrine tumor; SCA, serous cystadenoma; LECP, lymphoepithelial cyst; IPMN, intraductal papillary mucinous neoplasm; BD, branch duct; MD, main duct; SPN, solid pseudopapillary neoplasm.

aging features overlap with those of BD-IPMN [27]. Peripheral enhancement is variable, as are calcifications [4].

The aspirated fluid is described as clear. A few glandular cells and cells with squamous differentiation, probably correlating with squamous metaplasia of the duct, have been described [26].

Key Cytological Features
- Clear fluid
- Squamous metaplasia
- Glandular cells

Ancillary Testing
CEA may be elevated, which could lead to misclassification as an IPMN or MCN. *KRAS* and *GNAS* mutations should be absent if the cyst is lined by metaplastic or benign cuboidal epithelium. The absence of mutations does not rule out neoplasia.

Differential Diagnosis
Other cysts with inflammatory cellular contents. BD-IPMN may be in the differential. Retention cysts lack molecular alterations.

Pseudocyst
Pseudocysts lack a true epithelial lining and predominantly contain a mixture of pancreatic secretions, necrotic debris, and blood from resultant pancreatic enzyme-induced autodigestion of pancreatic parenchyma. Pseudocysts occur as the sequelae of acute pancreatitis, but also in the setting of chronic pancreatitis, postoperatively, or after pancreatic trauma [28]. Abdominal pain and early satiety are common presenting symptoms, with gastric outlet obstruction a potential risk. Thirty-three percent of pseudocysts are expected to resolve during the maturation period of 2–6 weeks [28]. Persistent pseudocysts can lead to complications such

as infection, hemorrhage, and rupture. Management depends on the size of the cyst, the location, and symptoms [28]. On imaging studies, pseudocysts are usually unilocular, with a very well-defined regular wall. Rim calcification may or may not be present. Any antecedent features of pancreatitis, such as inflammation, parenchymal calcification, and atrophy, will help clinch the diagnosis if present [4]. These may connect to the main pancreatic duct and internal debris may or may not be present. Histopathology shows a cyst lacking an epithelial cyst lining. The wall is composed of fibrous tissue with inflammatory cells. The cyst contains debris, pigment, and histiocytic inflammation.

The aspirated fluid is typically brown to red, granular, oily, and has an overall grungy appearance. Cytological features consist of cellular debris, inflammatory cells, hemosiderin-laden macrophages, and yellow pigment (Fig. 2) [29]. The yellow pigment is the defining cytological characteristic which can differentiate pseudocyst from other cysts. The background will lack thick extracellular mucin; however, contaminants from the gastrointestinal tract may be present. No cyst lining cells should be present. Aspirated gastric or duodenal epithelium may be the source of epithelia atypia in these cyst aspirates [29].

Key Cytological Features
- Abundant turbid fluid
- Macrophages, mixed inflammation
- Yellow pigment
- Lacks neoplastic epithelium

Ancillary Testing
Cyst fluid analysis shows a consistent elevation in amylase. CEA is usually low. In one study, the median CEA level was 41 ng/mL. However, a few patients had a CEA level >200 ng/mL [29]. Molecular mutations should be absent, although aspiration of adjacent intraepithelial neoplasia could lead to false positive results (pers. data).

Differential Diagnosis
While the cytological features are quite characteristic, ruling out abscess formation due to a secondary infection and discovery of a hidden adenocarcinoma should be emphasized.

Squamoid Cyst of Pancreatic Ducts
Squamoid cyst of the pancreatic ducts is a fairly recently described non-neoplastic cystic entity [30]. The cyst is lined by benign squamous epithelium. There is no established gender predominance and reported cases have occurred in pa-

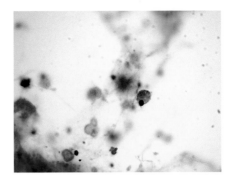

Fig. 2. Pseudocyst. Macrophages, debris, and background yellow pigment. Papanicolaou stain.

tients ranging from 50 to over 70 years old. Abdominal pain and mass-related symptoms are known to occur in association, or it is possible that these cysts can be incidentally found. A connection to the pancreatic ductal system is usually not seen.

The cytological features have been largely non-diagnostic according to a case series. Degenerated cells and histiocytes may comprise the background.

Key Cytological Features
- Acellular debris
- Lacks mucin
- Possibly squamous cells

Ancillary Testing
These have been reported to have elevated CEA levels [31]. The squamous component, if present, will be positive with markers of squamous differentiation, such as CK5/6, p63, and p40.

Differential Diagnosis
An elevated CEA may lead to a spurious diagnosis of mucinous cyst. If squamous epithelium is encountered, the differential diagnosis includes LECP, other cysts with a squamous lining, squamous metaplasia of the ductal system, and carcinomas with squamous differentiation.

Lymphoepithelial Cyst
LECP is rare, but when present it is most commonly seen in middle-aged men, with a male-to-female ratio of 4:1 [32]. Patients are usually asymptomatic but may present with abdominal pain, nausea, and anorexia. The cyst is squamous-lined, with underlying benign lymphoid tissue.

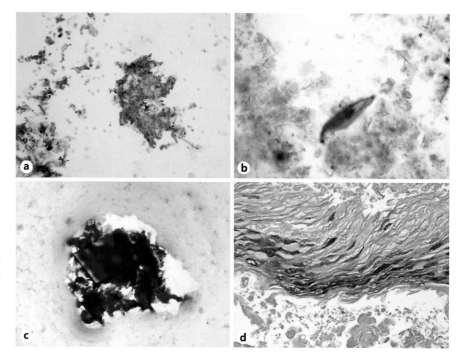

Fig. 3. Lymphoepithelial cyst. **a** Intermediate power showing anucleated squamous cells in aggregates. Papanicolaou stain. **b** Nucleated squamous cell in background debris. Papanicolaou stain. **c** Cholesterol crystal. Diff-Quik stain. **d** Intact granular layer in the cell block. HE stain.

The cytological features include nucleated and anucleated squamous cells and keratinous debris and cholesterol crystals (Fig. 3a–d) [33]. The background may consist of variable amounts of histiocytes and lymphocytes. Cyst aspirates are usually devoid of fluid.

Key Cytological Features
- Keratinous debris with anucleated and nucleated squamous cells
- Background lymphocytes and histiocytes
- With or without cholesterol crystals

Ancillary Testing
Due to these cysts appearing solid and commonly lacking fluid contents, biochemical analysis is not usually performed. If a CEA level is taken and noted to be elevated, caution should be exercised given the adjoining morphological characteristics [33, 34]. Molecular mutations should be absent.

Differential Diagnosis
Differential diagnoses include entities such as a dermoid cysts or splenic epidermoid cyst. The keratinous debris, when degenerated and without nuclei, can sometimes be mistaken for non-diagnostic amorphous cyst contents.

Foregut Cyst
Foregut cysts are rare congenital malformations considered to be a subgroup of duplication cysts. Foregut cysts are composed of a combination of epithelium from any of the foregut organs (tracheobronchial tree, esophagus, and gastrointestinal tract), and other tissues from those organs such as cartilage in bronchogenic cysts. There are a few reports of foregut cysts occurring in the pancreas. The cysts are defined according to the lining epithelium and surrounding structures. Ciliated foregut cysts are the simplest, lined by ciliated, columnar epithelium and a fibrous lining, lacking smooth muscle, and ciliated cysts are the most frequently reported in the literature occurring in the pancreas. The clinical presentation is variable, ranging from abdominal pain and pancreatitis to purely asymptomatic, as they can be incidental findings. Imaging-based differential diagnoses may be problematic due to considerable overlapping features with other pancreatic cystic lesions such as IPMN, MCN, and SPN.

Aspirated fluid is described as viscous and having mucin [35]. The CEA level has been reported as elevated [36, 37], and the background may contain mucin and cyst debris with amorphous material and macrophages [38, 39]. The diagnostic features are ciliated columnar cells and detached ciliary tufts (Fig. 4) [40]. Goblet cells can also be seen admixed with the associated epithelial fragments.

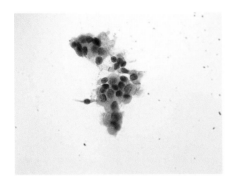

Fig. 4. Ciliated foregut cyst. Cluster of columnar cells with cilia. Papanicolaou stain.

Key Cytological Features
- Cystic fluid background with amorphous debris and macrophages
- Ciliated columnar cells and detached ciliary tufts
- No defined ancillary tests

Ancillary Testing
There are currently no particular, widely accepted ancillary studies to be performed. As noted, these have been reported with elevated CEA levels and amylase levels.

Differential Diagnosis
The main differential includes other cysts containing mucin, such as MCN and IPMN. Ciliated cells are characteristic of ciliated foregut cysts.

Neoplastic Cysts

Serous Cystadenoma
SCA is a benign neoplasm of the pancreas lined by small cuboidal cells containing glycogen. It has also been known by the synonyms microcystic cystadenoma and glycogen-rich cystadenoma. There have been rare reports of a malignant variant [41], but more recent data and review of the literature dispute the occurrence of truly malignant serous cystic neoplasms [42]. No deaths due to serous cystic neoplasms have been reported, and no features such as true invasion or metastases have been described. SCAs account for 1–2% of all pancreatic neoplasms [43].

SCAs occur more often in women than men, with a female-to-male ratio of 3:1. Depending on the study, the mean age is reported to be between the late 50s and 60s [41, 44]. A large single institutional review of 106 patients confirmed the increased incidence in women (75%) and a mean age of 61.5 years. The neoplasms occurred at an earlier age in women (59.2 years) compared to men (67.2 years) [44]. The majority of patients are now discovered incidentally. Presenting symptoms include abdominal pain, mass or fullness, jaundice, and fatigue and/or malaise. SCA occurs in patients with VHL disease [45], and there is an association with loss of heterozygosity on chromosome 3p25 and mutations in *VHL*.

The classic radiological imaging finding is that of a well-defined, microcystic or honeycomb mass with a central stellate scar and a starburst appearance due to calcifications. Other descriptions include "soap bubble" or "sponge-like." Only a small percentage of cases have this classic appearance [46, 47]. Other morphological variants include the macrocystic variant [48] or oligocystic variant [49] and the solid variant [42, 50], which mimics a neuroendocrine tumor on imaging. The risk of rupture is greatest when SCA is greater than 4 cm [44].

The tumors are composed of cysts lined by cuboidal cells with round, monomorphic nuclei. The surrounding stroma is fibrous and vascular. The cyst lining contains glycogen, which is demonstrated by periodic acid-Schiff (PAS) stain with and without diastase, with the diastase digesting the glycogen. The cells are positive with immunohistochemical evaluation for alpha-inhibin, MUC6, GLUT1, and vascular endothelial growth factor [51–53].

Molecular analysis shows alterations in the *VHL* gene and 3p deletions. These neoplasms lack the characteristic mutations of PDAC, including mutations in *KRAS* and *DPC4*, and mutations identified in other cystic neoplasms, such as *KRAS*, *GNAS*, and *RNF43* [54].

The aspirated fluid is thin, clear, and light brown or bloody. Aspirates are typically sparsely cellular. A careful search for cells is warranted, and a definite diagnosis may be rendered when the morphology fits the imaging appearance. The background is clean and granular, and lacks extracellular mucin, unless it is derived from contaminating mucin. The tumor cells form loose clusters or monolayered sheets, while the cells themselves are cuboidal with indistinct cell borders and a granular or clear cytoplasm. The cytoplasm is fragile and often the nuclei are stripped from the cytoplasm. The nuclei are round, small, and have indistinct nucleoli (Fig. 5a, b) [55, 56]. In a scantly cellular smear without diagnostic epithelium, hemosiderin-laden macrophages serve as surrogate markers of SCA as these neoplasms are vascular and bleed easily [57]. The diagnosis of SCA can be suggested when these are present and the imaging and PCF CEA and amylase levels are supportive.

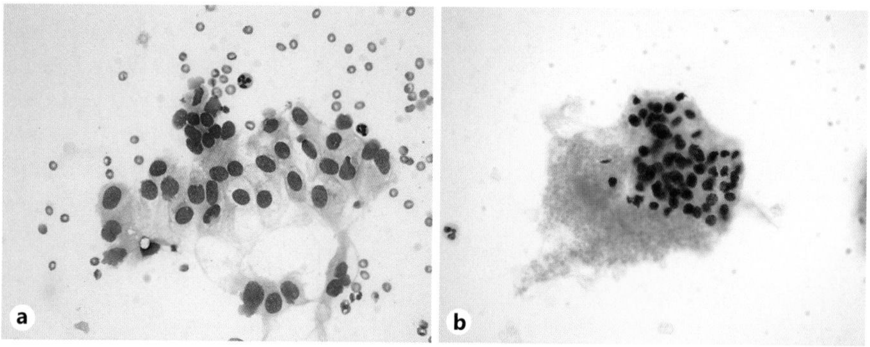

Fig. 5. SCA. **a** The cells are in a flat sheet. The cytoplasm is clear, with sharp borders. The nuclei are round to oval. **b** Cluster of neoplastic cells in a ThinPrep®. The nuclei are round, with smooth nuclear membranes and evenly distributed chromatin. ThinPrep®, Papanicolaou stain.

FNA samples are frequently non-diagnostic. Next-generation biopsy devices that collect small tissue fragments may improve the diagnosis of these lesions. At our cancer center, the advanced endoscopists have sampled two solid SCAs, which were previously non-diagnostic by FNA, using the Acquire™ needle (Boston Scientific, Boston, MA, USA). The biopsy obtained a core with small cysts surrounded by hyalinized, fibrous stroma with numerous capillaries. The neoplastic cells were small and cuboidal. PAS with and without diastase demonstrated cytoplasmic glycogen. The cells were positive for MUC6 and inhibin (Fig. 6a–e).

Key Cytological Features
- Scantly cellular smears with cells arranged in flat monolayered sheets or clusters
- Clean or bloody background lacking extracellular mucin (except for possible contamination)
- Uniform cuboidal cells with clear, finely vacuolated or granular cytoplasm
- Small, round nuclei with smooth nuclear membranes and inconspicuous nucleoli
- Hemosiderin-laden macrophages as a surrogate

Ancillary Studies
Biochemical analysis of cyst fluid will show low CEA and amylase levels. Molecular analysis will show mutations in the *VHL* gene [16]. The neoplastic cells are positive with MUC6 and inhibin.

Differentia Diagnosis
When epithelium is present, the key differential diagnosis is with benign ductal cells, and neoplasms with a monomorphic appearance, such as PanNET. Benign ductal epithelium lacks the clear cytoplasm, and the cells are arranged in monolayered sheets. PanNET has a variable cytoplasm and round nuclei with salt and pepper chromatin. PCF CEA,

amylase, and molecular analysis and immunohistochemistry are helpful. If yellow pigment is absent, and only hemosiderin-laden macrophages are present, the diagnosis of pseudocyst is unlikely.

Preinvasive Precursors
MCN and IPMN are both precursor lesions to PDAC. They have unique clinicopathological features, but similar cytological findings. The role of EUS-FNA is to identify lesions as being mucinous, and to further stratify them according to the risk of underlying high-grade dysplasia or malignancy.

Mucinous Cystic Neoplasm
MCN is an epithelial, cystic neoplasm lined by columnar, mucinous epithelium with subepithelial ovarian-type stroma. The majority of patients are female (95–98%) [58, 59], and the average patient age at presentation is between 40 and 50 years [43]. The majority present with an incidentally discovered mass, or vague abdominal symptoms, although some may present with acute pancreatitis or a palpable mass [60]. Most patients are curable with complete resection, and patients who undergo resection have 100% 5-year survival in the absence of an invasive component [61]. Patients with an invasive component have a 57% 5-year survival [59], although in another series it was 26% [58]. Survival depends on the size and extent of the invasive component [58, 59]. Patients with an invasive component tend to be older by 10–11 years [59].

The typical imaging presentation is that of a single cyst, most often located in the distal pancreas [60]. They should not have a communication with the pancreatic ductal system, but occasionally a communication is reported. The mass may have separations and multiple locules. The imaging differential diagnosis will be the macrocystic variant of SCA. Peripheral calcifications may be noted in about 20%. Thick septations, internal papillary projections, and a mural

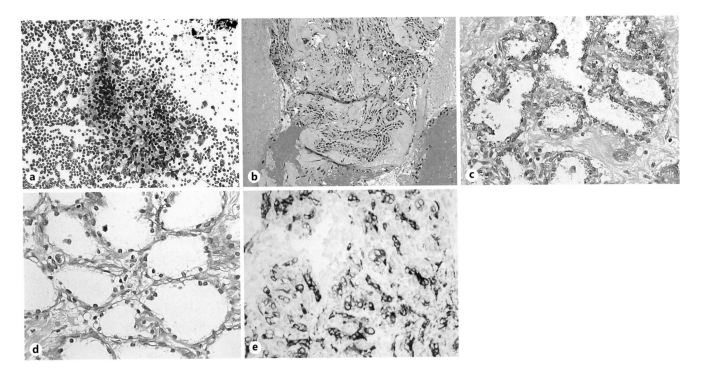

Fig. 6. SCA, solid variant. This sample was obtained using one of the next-generation biopsy devices, the Acquire needle biopsy (Boston Scientific). Previous aspirates had been non-diagnostic. **a** A flat sheet of epithelium, with round, monomorphous nuclei is characteristic for on-site adequacy. **b** Core fragment with microcysts lined by flattened cuboidal epithelium, surrounded by hyalinized, fibrotic stroma with small capillaries. HE stain. PAS shows cytoplasmic granules in the neoplastic cyst lining cells (**c**; cell block, PAS stain) which is digested by diastase, confirming the presence of glycogen (**d**; cell block, dPAS stain). **e** The neoplastic cells are positive for MUC6. Cell block, immunoperoxidase stain.

nodule are features associated with an invasive component [60]. Also, larger size, >4 cm, is also associated with a greater risk of an invasive component [59].

Histologically, the neoplasms are composed of epithelial, columnar mucinous epithelium surrounded by ovarian-type stroma (Fig. 7a, b). The cells resemble pseudopyloric, foveolar, small intestinal and large intestinal epithelium with interspersed neuroendocrine cells. The lining epithelium is graded according to the grade of dysplasia: low or high grade, according to the WHO 2019 classification. The invasive component is most frequently the usual ductal type, although papillary morphologies and undifferentiated morphology are also associated with MCN [58, 60]. The epithelium expresses CK7, CK18, and CK19, epithelial membrane antigen, CEA, and MUC5AC. The invasive component may express MUC1. Synaptophysin and chromogranin will identify the neuroendocrine cells. The stroma is positive for vimentin, smooth muscle actin, estrogen receptor, and progesterone receptor.

Analysis of molecular alterations reveals mutations in *KRAS* codon 12. Other mutations include *RNF43*. MCN with high-grade dysplasia may show alterations in *TP53*. Mutation in *SMAD4* is a feature of invasive carcinoma and can be identified by using immunohistochemistry for SMAD4, which will show loss of protein expression [60]. MCNs do not show mutations in *GNAS*.

Aspirated cyst fluid is viscous. The background typically contains thick mucin. A varying number of neoplastic cells are present. The degree of atypia depends on the grade of cyst lining dysplasia.

Key Cytological Features
- Viscous cyst fluid
- Thick background mucin
- Mucinous neoplastic epithelium with varying degrees of atypia (see the description of low-grade and high-grade epithelial atypia in the following section, Intraductal Papillary Mucinous Neoplasm)

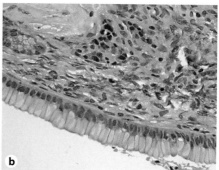

Fig. 7. MCN. **a** Low-power image showing a cyst lined by columnar, mucinous epithelium. The stroma is cellular and ovarian type. HE stain. **b** This neoplasm has low-grade dysplasia. The nuclei remain basally located, and the cytoplasm is tall and columnar with mucin. HE stain.

Ancillary studies

The CEA is elevated, and the amylase is variable. These cysts harbor mutations in *KRAS* but lack mutations in *GNAS*.

Differential Diagnosis

The cytological features of MCN overlap with those of IPMN, and the two cannot be differentiated on the basis of cytology alone, since the ovarian-type stroma is not sampled by the FNA. SCA is excluded by the elevated CEA, and the presence of thick, background mucin. These cysts lack the anucleated and nucleated debris seen in LECP, another cyst that may produce an elevated CEA.

Intraductal Papillary Mucinous Neoplasm

IPMN is a neoplastic proliferation replacing pancreatic ducts with mucinous, papillary neoplastic epithelium. It replaces the main pancreatic duct or its side branches, or both. The mean age at presentation is 63 years, and there is a slight predominance in men [1]. Most patients are asymptomatic and their cyst is discovered incidentally. Presenting symptoms include those related to chronic pancreatitis secondary to duct obstruction, and may have been present for many years.

IPMNs are classified based on the imaging studies as main pancreatic duct type (MD-IPMN), branch-duct type (BD-IPMN), or combined type (C-IPMN) when they involve both. MD-IPMN presents as dilation of the main pancreatic duct, more commonly in the head of the pancreas, but sometimes throughout the entire pancreas. A diagnostic feature of MD-IPMN in the head of the pancreas on endoscopy is a patulous, "fish-mouth"-appearing Ampulla of Vater, from which abundant mucus extrudes. BD-IPMN may be single, unilocular cysts, or multiple, bunched up clusters of cysts. On imaging, a connection to the main pancreatic duct and/or multiple cysts are suggestive of BD-IPMN.

Patient management is dictated by the risk of malignancy. The revised Fukuoka guidelines, published in 2017, are used to guide the management of patients with IPMN [62]. The indications for immediate surgery are obstructive jaundice, an enhancing mural nodule >5 mm, and main pancreatic duct dilation >10 mm. Patients with "worrisome" features are referred to EUS-FNA. Pancreatitis is a worrisome clinical feature. Worrisome imaging features include: (1) cyst >3 cm, (2) enhancing mural nodule <5 mm, (3) thickened/enhancing cyst walls, (4) main duct size 5–9 mm, (5) an abrupt change in the caliber of pancreatic duct with distal pancreatic atrophy, (6) lymphadenopathy, and (7) an increased serum level of CA19-9 and cyst growth rate >5 mm/2 years. If EUS shows a definite mural nodule 5 mm or greater, or suggests main pancreatic duct involvement, or FNA cytology is suspicious or positive for malignancy, the patient should be referred for surgical consultation. The patient may be referred for surveillance if these criteria are lacking.

The role of the pathologist assessing EUS-FNA cytology samples from pancreatic cysts with worrisome features is to detect cells indicative of high-grade dysplasia or adenocarcinoma. High-grade epithelial atypia recognizes epithelial cells with atypia that is qualitatively and quantitatively insufficient for a diagnosis of malignancy [62], but that is predictive of high-grade dysplasia or adenocarcinoma [63].

IPMN is a mucin-producing neoplasm of the pancreatic ductal system, variably forming papillae. The neoplastic epithelium has been characterized into three epithelial types: intestinal, pancreatobiliary, and gastric. These are defined by morphology and their mucin (MUC) profiles. All express MUC5AC and CK7/CK8/CK18/CK19. The intestinal type (Fig. 8a) shows villous papillae, with basophilic cytoplasm, enlarged oval nuclei, pseudostratification, and hyperchromatic nuclei. The intestinal type expresses MUC2, CDX2, and CK20, and is negative for MUC1 (Fig. 8b–d). The pan-

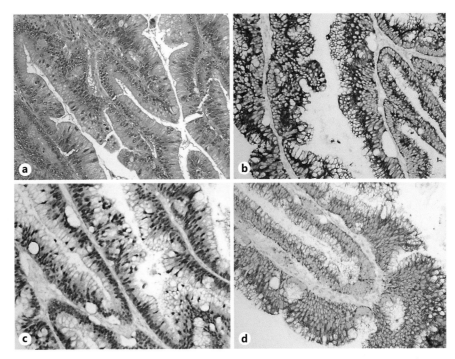

Fig. 8. IPMN, intestinal type. **a** Papillary proliferation lined by columnar, mucinous epithelium composed of pseudostratified, columnar epithelium, with elongated cigar-shaped nuclei. HE stain. The cells are positive for MUC2 (**b**), CDX2 (**c**) and MUC5 (**d**). Immunoperoxidase stain.

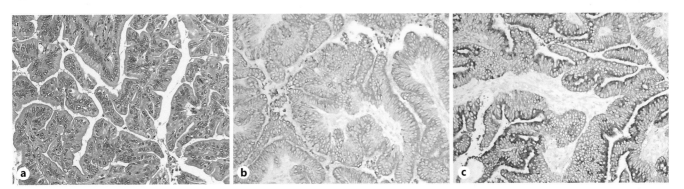

Fig. 9. IPMN, pancreatobiliary type. **a** Short papillae lined by cuboidal cells with eosinophilic cytoplasm. The nuclei are round with vesicular chromatin and nucleoli. HE stain. MUC1 (**b**) and MUC5 (**c**). Immunoperoxidase stain.

creatobiliary type shows thin, branching papillae, moderate amphophilic cytoplasm, and enlarged, hyperchromatic nuclei sometimes with nucleoli. They express MUC1 and MUC6 and are negative for MUC2 and CDX2 (Fig. 9a–c). The gastric foveolar subtype shows thick, finger-like papillae or flat epithelium. The cytoplasm is typically eosinophilic, and the nuclei basally located. The gastric foveolar type expresses MUC5AC (Fig. 10a, b). Subtyping of IPMN on small biopsies is impractical and does not add to patient management.

The neoplastic epithelium shows increasing grades of dysplasia classified as a two-tiered system: low-grade dys-

plasia and high-grade dysplasia [2]. The former intermediate-grade category is now included in the low-grade dysplasia group. Low-grade dysplasia is characterized by tall columnar mucin containing epithelium with minimal to mild nuclear atypia, basally located nuclei, and with or without papillary projections or mitoses [2]. High-grade dysplasia is characterized by loss of polarity, an increased nuclear-to-cytoplasmic ratio, tufting, prominent nucleoli, numerous mitoses, and nuclear pleomorphism. Figure 11a–c shows the histopathology with grades of dysplasia.

The Baltimore consensus conference recommended reporting the dysplasia using a two-tiered system, incorporat-

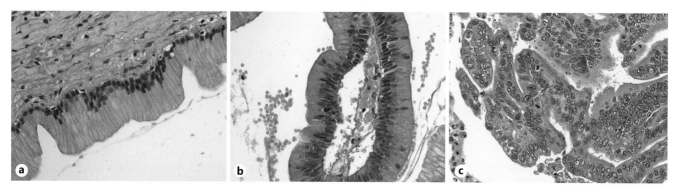

Fig. 10. IPMN, gastric foveolar type. **a** Cyst lined by columnar mucinous epithelium with basally located nuclei. The nuclei have minimal atypia. HE stain. **b** The cytoplasm is diffusely positive for MUC5. Immunoperoxidase stain.

Fig. 11. IPMN, grades of dysplasia. **a** Low-grade dysplasia. Tall, columnar epithelium with basally located, small nuclei. HE stain. **b** Low-grade dysplasia. The nuclei are pseudostratified and hyperchromatic. There are no mitoses identified. This would have been classified as intermediate dysplasia in the previous classification. HE stain. **c** High-grade dysplasia. The cells have lost their polarity. There is an increased N:C ratio, the nuclear are vesicular, and there are prominent nucleoli. HE stain.

ing low-grade and moderate-grade dysplasia into the low-grade dysplasia category, and leaving only high-grade dysplasia in the high-grade category [64].

Aspiration of IPMN obtains thick, viscous fluid, and this gross fluid finding serves as the first indication of a mucinous cyst. The aspirate smears show mucin, with or without neoplastic epithelium. The classic appearance of mucin from IPMN is thick, pink, colloid-like material covering the smear, but it may also be thin and watery (Fig. 12a–c). The mucin may also be thick, inspissated, and fan-like or fibrillary in appearance (Fig. 13).

If neoplastic cells are present, they need to be evaluated for the architectural and cytological features in order to determine the possible grade of dysplasia and risk of malignancy. A practical approach, and one that is in line with the Baltimore consensus [64] and patient management guidelines [62], is to group the dysplasia in the cytology smears into two categories: low-grade and high-grade cytological atypia. Low-grade cytological atypia incorporates low-grade and intermediate-grade dysplasia, and high-grade cytological atypia incorporates high-grade dysplasia and invasive adenocarcinoma [65]. Cells with low-grade epithelial atypia are the size of enterocytes (12 μ), have a low nuclear-to-cytoplasmic ratio, and minimal nuclear atypia (Fig. 14a–e). High-grade epithelial atypia is defined as cells that are smaller than enterocytes, with an increased nuclear-to-cytoplasmic ratio, nuclear membrane irregularities, and hyperchromasia (Fig. 15a–e). Necrosis is the only feature that predicts invasion.

Key Cytological Features
- Background mucin
  Thick, colloid-like mucin with or without mucinous epithelium
  Thin, watery mucin
  Inspissated material

Centeno/Thomas

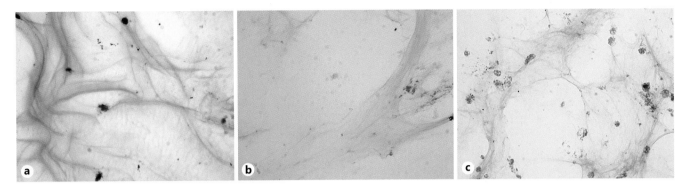

Fig. 12. IPMN and MCN, background mucin. **a** Thick, pink, colloid-type background mucin. Papanicolaou stain. **b** Watery-appearing background mucin with some debris. Papanicolaou stain. **c** Thick mucin and oncotic cells in a liquid-based cytology specimen. ThinPrep®, Papanicolaou stain.

- Glandular epithelium with:
  Low-grade epithelial atypia
- Cells the size of an enterocyte (12 μm) or larger
- Retained N:C ratio
- Minimal nuclear membrane irregularities
- Euchromatic, rarely hypo- or hyperchromatic
- Columnar appearance with cytoplasmic mucin filling the cytoplasmic compartment
  High-grade epithelial atypia
- Single intact cells (<12 μm duodenal enterocyte)
- Cell doublets and small cell clusters, cellular papillary groups
- Nuclear membrane irregularity
- Significantly increased N:C ratio
- Abnormal chromatin (hypo- or hyperchromatic)
- Background necrosis (invasion)

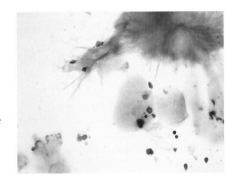

Fig. 13. IPMN. Inspissated background material, with fibrillary edges and a calcification.

Ancillary Testing

Almost all IPMNs have either *KRAS, RNF43*, or *GNAS* mutation. The detection of a *KRAS* mutation supports the presence of a neoplastic mucinous cyst and the detection of a *GNAS* mutation distinguishes an IPMN from an MCN. *KRAS* mutations predominantly occur on codons 12 and 13; however, more than one mutant clone of *KRAS* may occur in a single IPMN cyst, and distinct IPMN cysts often have different *KRAS* mutations. *GNAS* mutations appear to occur only at codon 201, and this mutation seems to be specific to IPMNs and the invasive carcinomas arising from them.

Differential Diagnosis of Mucinous Cysts

Other entities associated with extracellular mucin; these include gastric or duodenal contaminant, and mucinous carcinoma. The mucin from gastric and duodenal contaminant

lacks oncotic cells and histiocytes, and is thin and watery. Gastric foveolar epithelium has cupped-shaped mucin (Fig. 16) rather than mucin that extends to nuclei (Fig. 14a). The groups are hypercellular in neoplastic epithelium with crowded nuclei with atypia (Fig. 17a, b), whereas the foveolar epithelium is relatively flat (Fig. 18). The nuclei may be stripped and embedded in the mucin.

Mucinous carcinoma has a combination of characteristic, thick background mucin, and malignant glandular epithelium. In the absence of a confirmed mass, it may be difficult to definitively differentiate mucinous carcinoma from high-grade dysplasia.

Intraductal Oncocytic Papillary Neoplasms

Intraductal oncocytic papillary neoplasm (IOPN) is a grossly cystic neoplasm of the pancreas lined by oncocytic glandular epithelium [2]. The age range is 36–87 years (mean 59 years) and they are more common in females. IOPN are grossly uni-

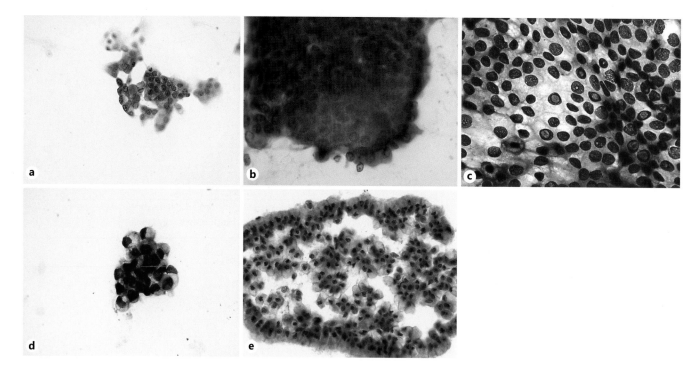

Fig. 14. IPMN, Low-grade epithelial atypia. **a** Columnar cells with abundant cytoplasmic mucin, basally located nuclei with minimal atypia. The cells are larger than an enterocyte. Papanicolaou stain. **b** Group with nuclear overlapping. The cells retain their nuclear-to-cytoplasmic ratio. The nuclear membranes have minimal atypia. The chromatin is pale. Papanicolaou stain. **c** These cells are in a sheet, with irregularly distributed nuclei. The cells still have abundant cytoplasm. Prominent intranuclear inclusions are identified. Diff-Quik stain. **d** Micropapillary cluster. The cells have cytoplasmic mucin and a low nuclear-to-cytoplasmic ratio. The nuclei are angulated. Diff-Quik stain. **e** Columnar, mucinous epithelium with minimal nuclear atypia. The nuclei are basally located. ThinPrep®, Papanicolaou stain.

locular or multilocular cystic masses. IOPN has complex and arborizing papilla with delicate fibrovascular cores. The papillae are lined by oncocytic cells with interspersed goblet cells. The lining epithelium may show a cribriform or solid growth pattern [2]. Most of the neoplastic cells are oncocytic, with few interspersed goblet cells. The lining epithelium may be mixed with the usual types of IPMN epithelium.

Originally considered to possibly be a variant of IPMN, these are now considered a distinct entity, based on immunophenotypic and molecular analysis. Studies report conflicting results about the presence of *KRAS* and *GNAS* alterations, with some reporting these neoplasms as lacking these mutations, and others reporting their presence. Analysis of a series of IOPN showed that the areas with pure oncocytic morphology lacked mutations in *KRAS* and *GNAS*. Instead, these areas have alterations in *ARHGAP26*, *ASXL1*, *EPHA8*, and *ERBB4* genes [66].

Smears are typically hypercellular, with well-formed clusters of cells. The cells have oncocytic cytoplasm with round nuclei with prominent nucleoli (Fig. 19a). They may

have background mucin and interspersed cells with mucin. These may be mistaken for PDAC on cytology, and imaging may be confusing, as they may appear as a solid mass. The cell block may show fibrovascular cores lined by oncocytic cells (Fig. 19b).

Key Cytological Features
• Cellular smears
• Oncocytic cytoplasm
• Round nuclei with prominent nucleoli

Ancillary Testing
IOPN is positive for MUC6, MUC1, and MUC5AC. The goblet cells are positive for MUC2, CDX2, and CK20. The presence of goblet cells interspersed with oncocytic cells differentiates this from pancreatobiliary IPMN. The oncocytic cells express anti-mitochondrial antibodies when assessed by immunohistochemistry. These may show mutations in *KRAS* if associated with other typical IPMN; however, as described, they have unique molecular alterations.

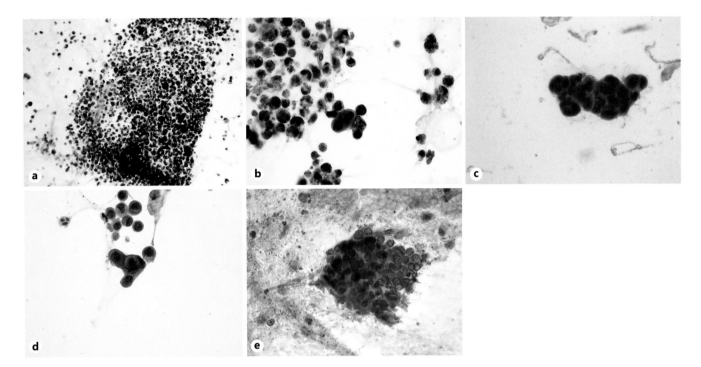

Fig. 15. IPMN, high-grade epithelial atypia. **a** Intermediate power shows abundant oncotic debris obscuring the neoplastic cells. ThinPrep®, Papanicolaou stain. **b** The neoplastic cells are small, with a high nuclear-to-cytoplasmic ratio, hyperchromasia, and irregular nuclear membranes. ThinPrep®, Papanicolaou stain. **c** Nuclear overlap with nuclear enlargement, and an increased nuclear-to-cytoplasmic ratio. Papanicolaou stain. **d** Small cells, with a high nuclear-to-cytoplasmic ratio, and hyperchromasia. Papanicolaou stain. **e** A crowded group, with nuclear overlapping and anisonucleosis. There is background debris, suggestive of necrosis. This group has features suspicious for invasion. Papanicolaou stain.

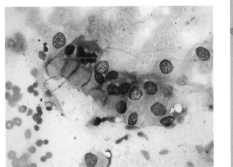

Fig. 16. Gastric epithelium with cup-shaped mucin. Diff-Quik stain.

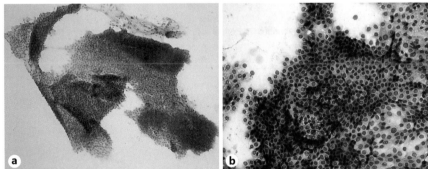

Fig. 17. IPMN. **a** The neoplastic epithelium may form large, hypercellular, folded sheets. The hypercellularity and crowding distinguishes this from foveolar epithelium. Papanicolaou stain. **b** The neoplastic sheets show loss of polarity. Binucleation, subtle anisonucleosis, and nuclear angulation are evident. Diff-Quik stain.

Differential Diagnosis

The main differential diagnosis is with other lesions with oncocytic cytoplasm, in particular oncocytic PanNET. Immunohistochemistry for neuroendocrine markers will assist with this diagnosis. Acinar cell carcinoma may also have an oncocytic cytoplasm, although this is uncommon [67].

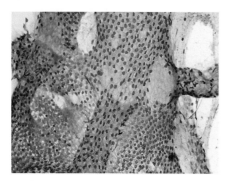

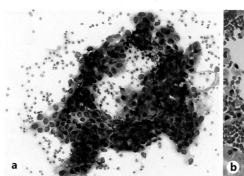

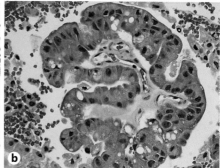

Fig. 18. Benign gastric epithelium arranged in a flat sheet, with uniformly spaced cells. The nuclei and cytoplasmic shapes are uniform in appearance. There is no nuclear crowding. Diff-Quik stain.

Fig. 19. IOPN. **a** Flat sheet of neoplastic cells with sharp borders and abundant cytoplasm, the nuclei are round and uniform. **b** Papillary groups with a central fibrovascular core and oncocytic cells clearly identified on the cell block. HE stain.

20

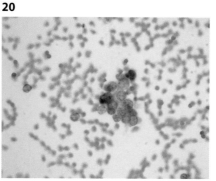

21

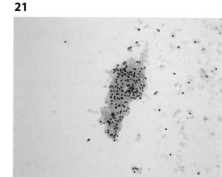

Fig. 20. Cystic PanNET. Cluster of cells with an increased nuclear-to-cytoplasmic ratio, scant cytoplasm, round nuclei, smooth nuclear membranes, and salt and pepper chromatin. Papanicolaou stain.

Fig. 21. Lymphangioma. The aspirate contains a mixed population of lymphocytes and lacks background mucin, pigment, and epithelial cells. ThinPrep®, Papanicolaou stain.

Solid Neoplasms with Cystic Degeneration

Any solid neoplasm may undergo cystic degeneration and present as a cystic mass on imaging. The two most relevant to this discussion are SPN and PanNET. The clinical, imaging, cytological, and ancillary studies for each are discussed in the chapter by Dhillon [this vol., pp. 92–108] on non-ductal neoplasms. SPN is known to be in the differential diagnosis of cystic masses and presents as a solid and cystic mass on imaging.

Cystic PanNET may present as a unilocular, completely cystic mass, mimicking MCN. The aspirated cells will appear to have a high nuclear-to-cytoplasmic ratio, suggesting high-grade epithelial atypia. The cytological features are as described for PanNET (Fig. 20). The immunophenotype remains the same. These cysts will have low CEA and amylase, and lack mutations in *KRAS, GNAS, VHL, CTNBB1,* and other mutations associated with cystic neoplasms of the pancreas [68].

Non-Epithelial Cysts

Lymphangioma

Lymphangiomas of the pancreas are rare, benign neoplasms, occurring either in the pancreatic parenchyma, adjacent to the pancreas, or connected to the pancreas by a pedicle [69–71]. They may be cystic or cavernous. These have a female predilection, and a wide age range (2–61 years, mean 29). Patients may present with non-specific symptoms, such as abdominal pain or nausea and vomiting. On ultrasound imaging, they present as anechoic or hypoechoic fluid-filled masses that are multicystic. CT imaging will show a well-circumscribed, homogenous, septate cystic mass in or adjacent to the pancreas. The prognosis is excellent.

FNA obtains yellow, straw-colored, turbid, occasionally white and watery, non-mucinous fluid. This chylous fluid is filled with small mature lymphocytes (Fig. 21) [72].

Key Cytological Features
• Small mature-appearing lymphocytes
• No epithelial cells
• Non-mucinous background

Ancillary Studies
CEA levels are low. The amylase level may show mild elevation in the low thousands, which could suggest the diagnosis of pseudocyst. Immunohistochemistry for D2-40 highlights the endothelial cells lining the lymphatic spaces. This will lack mutations associated with cystic neoplasms.

Differential Diagnosis
The differential diagnosis includes other cysts. The finding of mature lymphocytes and the absence of yellow pigment and macrophages excludes pseudocyst. An undersampled SCA could be in the differential diagnosis. The lack of mucin and the low CEA exclude MCN or IPMN.

Reporting of Pancreatic Cysts

The Papanicolaou Society of Cytopathology (PSC) Terminology system for pancreatobiliary cytology specimens, reviewed in the chapter by Dhillon [this vol., pp. 1–15], provides guidelines for the interpreting and reporting of PCF, which includes criteria for the identification of mucinous cysts. The system created six reporting categories: non-diagnostic, negative (for malignancy), atypical, neoplastic, suspicious (for malignancy), and positive/malignant [73]. These categories are for use in laboratories where the information system requires a diagnostic category for reporting cytology specimens. A key tenet of the system is that correlation of the clinical, imaging, and ancillary findings is necessary for determining the adequacy of a sample and formulating an interpretation. Using this system, a PCF is nondiagnostic if the sample volume is insufficient for processing and evaluation, or if it only yields normal pancreatic elements, gastrointestinal contaminant, or an acellular cyst fluid lacking background mucin, which is insufficient for ancillary testing.

Cysts without any risk for progression to malignancy are categorized as negative. PCF from pseudocysts, lymphoepithelial cyst, or lymphangioma would be categorized as negative.

The neoplastic category is further subdivided into neoplastic benign and neoplastic other. SCA is classified as neoplastic benign. IPMN and MCN are classified as neoplastic other, since they are preinvasive precursors. Any cyst classified as mucinous, based on the presence of background mucin, CEA levels, or *KRAS* or *GNAS* mutations, is categorized as neoplastic other [73]. When diagnostic epithelium is not identified, the interpretation should include a description of the findings. The comment should correlate the morphological findings with the imaging findings and CEA and amylase levels. Since the molecular results are typically not available at the same time as those of cytology, CEA, and amylase, the results of these may be added in an addendum, and used to provide a more definitive interpretation. It is never acceptable to interpret the cytology of a pancreatic cyst as consistent with the cyst contents.

Disclosure Statement

The authors have no conflicts of interest to disclose.

References

1 Hruban RH, Pitman MB, Klimstra DS: Tumors of the Pancreas. AFIP Atlas of Tumor Pathology. Silver Spring, American Registry of Pathology, 2007.
2 Gill AJ, Klimstra DS, Lam AK, Washington MK: 10 Tumours of the Pancreas; in WHO Classification of Tumours Editorial Board (ed): Digestive System Tumours. WHO Classification of Tumours, ed 5. Lyon, IARC, 2019, pp 295–372.
3 Fernandez-del Castillo C, Targarona J, Thayer SP, Rattner DW, Brugge WR, Warshaw AL: Incidental pancreatic cysts: clinicopathologic characteristics and comparison with symptomatic patients. Arch Surg 2003;138:427–434.
4 Sureka B, Bihari C, Arora A, Agrawal N, Bharathy KG, Jamwal KD, Mittal MK, Chattopadhyay TK: Imaging paradigm of cystic lesions in pancreas. J Pancreas 2016;17:452–465.
5 Brugge WR, Lewandrowski K, Lee-Lewandrowski E, Centeno BA, Szydlo T, Regan S, del Castillo CF, Warshaw AL: Diagnosis of pancreatic cystic neoplasms: a report of the cooperative pancreatic cyst study. Gastroenterology 2004;126:1330–1336.
6 van der Waaij LA, van Dullemen HM, Porte RJ: Cyst fluid analysis in the differential diagnosis of pancreatic cystic lesions: a pooled analysis. Gastrointest Endosc 2005;62:383–389.
7 Soyer OM, Baran B, Ormeci AC, Sahin D, Gokturk S, Evirgen S, Basar R, Firat P, Akyuz F, Demir K, Besisik F, Kaymakoglu S, Karaca C: Role of biochemistry and cytological analysis of cyst fluid for the differential diagnosis of pancreatic cysts: a retrospective cohort study. Medicine 2017;96:e5513.
8 Moris M, Raimondo M, Woodward TA, Skinner V, Arcidiacono PG, Petrone MC, De Angelis C, Manfre S, Fusaroli P, Asbun H, Stauffer J, Wallace MB: Diagnostic accuracy of endoscopic ultrasound-guided fine-needle aspiration cytology, carcinoembryonic antigen, and amylase in intraductal papillary mucinous neoplasm. Pancreas 2016;45:870–875.

9   Shami VM, Sundaram V, Stelow EB, Conaway M, Moskaluk CA, White GE, Adams RB, Yeaton P, Kahaleh M: The level of carcinoembryonic antigen and the presence of mucin as predictors of cystic pancreatic mucinous neoplasia. Pancreas 2007;34:466–469.

10 Park WG, Mascarenhas R, Palaez-Luna M, Smyrk TC, O'Kane D, Clain JE, Levy MJ, Pearson RK, Petersen BT, Topazian MD, Vege SS, Chari ST: Diagnostic performance of cyst fluid carcinoembryonic antigen and amylase in histologically confirmed pancreatic cysts. Pancreas 2011;40:42–45.

11 Cizginer S, Turner BG, Bilge AR, Karaca C, Pitman MB, Brugge WR: Cyst fluid carcinoembryonic antigen is an accurate diagnostic marker of pancreatic mucinous cysts. Pancreas 2011;40: 1024–1028.

12 Thornton GD, McPhail MJ, Nayagam S, Hewitt MJ, Vlavianos P, Monahan KJ: Endoscopic ultrasound guided fine needle aspiration for the diagnosis of pancreatic cystic neoplasms: a meta-analysis. Pancreatology 2013;13:48–57.

13 Das KK, Xiao H, Geng X, Fernandez-Del-Castillo C, Morales-Oyarvide V, Daglilar E, Forcione DG, Bounds BC, Brugge WR, Pitman MB, Mino-Kenudson M, Das KM: mAb Das-1 is specific for high-risk and malignant intraductal papillary mucinous neoplasm (IPMN). Gut 2014;63:1626–1634.

14 Das KK, Geng X, Brown JW, Morales-Oyarvide V, Huynh T, Pergolini I, Pitman MB, Ferrone C, Al Efishat M, Haviland D, Thompson E, Wolfgang C, Lennon AM, Allen P, Lillemoe KD, Fields RC, Hawkins WG, Liu J, Castillo CF, Das KM, Mino-Kenudson M: Cross validation of the monoclonal antibody Das-1 in identification of high-risk mucinous pancreatic cystic lesions. Gastroenterology 2019;157:720–730.e2.

15 Misdraji J, Centeno BA, Pitman MB: Ancillary tests in the diagnosis of liver and pancreatic neoplasms. Cancer Cytopathol 2018;126(suppl 8): 672–690.

16 Wu J, Jiao Y, Dal Molin M, Maitra A, de Wilde RF, Wood LD, Eshleman JR, Goggins MG, Wolfgang CL, Canto MI, Schulick RD, Edil BH, Choti MA, Adsay V, Klimstra DS, Offerhaus GJ, Klein AP, Kopelovich L, Carter H, Karchin R, Allen PJ, Schmidt CM, Naito Y, Diaz LA Jr, Kinzler KW, Papadopoulos N, Hruban RH, Vogelstein B: Whole-exome sequencing of neoplastic cysts of the pancreas reveals recurrent mutations in components of ubiquitin-dependent pathways. Proc Natl Acad Sci USA 2011;108:21188–21193.

17 Furukawa T, Kuboki Y, Tanji E, Yoshida S, Hatori T, Yamamoto M, Shibata N, Shimizu K, Kamatani N, Shiratori K: Whole-exome sequencing uncovers frequent GNAS mutations in intraductal papillary mucinous neoplasms of the pancreas. Sci Rep 2011;1:161.

18 Wu J, Matthaei H, Maitra A, Dal Molin M, Wood LD, Eshleman JR, Goggins M, Canto MI, Schulick RD, Edil BH, Wolfgang CL, Klein AP, Diaz LA Jr, Allen PJ, Schmidt CM, Kinzler KW, Papadopoulos N, Hruban RH, Vogelstein B: Recurrent GNAS mutations define an unexpected pathway for pancreatic cyst development. Sci Transl Med 2011;3: 92ra66.

19 Al-Haddad MA, Kowalski T, Siddiqui A, Mertz HR, Mallat D, Haddad N, Malhotra N, Sadowski B, Lybik MJ, Patel SN, Okoh E, Rosenkranz L, Karasik M, Golioto M, Linder J, Catalano MF: Integrated molecular pathology accurately determines the malignant potential of pancreatic cysts. Endoscopy 2015;47:136–142.

20 Rosenbaum MW, Jones M, Dudley JC, Le LP, Iafrate AJ, Pitman MB: Next-generation sequencing adds value to the preoperative diagnosis of pancreatic cysts. Cancer Cytopathol 2017;125: 41–47.

21 Nikiforova MN, Khalid A, Fasanella KE, McGrath KM, Brand RE, Chennat JS, Slivka A, Zeh HJ, Zureikat AH, Krasinskas AM, Ohori NP, Schoedel KE, Navina S, Mantha GS, Pai RK, Singhi AD: Integration of KRAS testing in the diagnosis of pancreatic cystic lesions: a clinical experience of 618 pancreatic cysts. Mod Pathol 2013;26:1478–1487.

22 Singhi AD, Nikiforova MN, Fasanella KE, McGrath KM, Pai RK, Ohori NP, Bartholow TL, Brand RE, Chennat JS, Lu X, Papachristou GI, Slivka A, Zeh HJ, Zureikat AH, Lee KK, Tsung A, Mantha GS, Khalid A: Preoperative GNAS and KRAS testing in the diagnosis of pancreatic mucinous cysts. Clin Cancer Res 2014;20:4381–4389.

23 Singhi AD, McGrath K, Brand RE, Khalid A, Zeh HJ, Chennat JS, Fasanella KE, Papachristou GI, Slivka A, Bartlett DL, Dasyam AK, Hogg M, Lee KK, Marsh JW, Monaco SE, Ohori NP, Pingpank JF, Tsung A, Zureikat AH, Wald AI, Nikiforova MN: Preoperative next-generation sequencing of pancreatic cyst fluid is highly accurate in cyst classification and detection of advanced neoplasia. Gut 2018;67:2131–2141.

24 Springer S, Wang Y, Dal Molin M, Masica DL, Jiao Y, Kinde I, et al: A combination of molecular markers and clinical features improve the classification of pancreatic cysts. Gastroenterology 2015; 149:1501–1510.

25 Kloppel G: Pseudocysts and other non-neoplastic cysts of the pancreas. Semin Diagn Pathol 2000; 17:7–15.

26 Ren F, Zuo C, Chen G, Wang J, Lu J, Shao C, Hao X: Pancreatic retention cyst: multi-modality imaging findings and review of the literature. Abdom Imaging 2013;38:818–826.

27 Goh BK, Tan YM, Chung YF, Chow PK, Ong HS, Lim DT, Wong WK, Ooi LL: Non-neoplastic cystic and cystic-like lesions of the pancreas: may mimic pancreatic cystic neoplasms. ANZ J Surg 2006;76: 325–331.

28 Pan G, Wan MH, Xie KL, Li W, Hu WM, Liu XB, Tang WF, Wu H: Classification and Management of Pancreatic Pseudocysts. Medicine 2015; 94:e960.

29 Gonzalez Obeso E, Murphy E, Brugge W, Deshpande V: Pseudocyst of the pancreas: the role of cytology and special stains for mucin. Cancer 2009;117:101–107.

30 Othman M, Basturk O, Groisman G, Krasinskas A, Adsay NV: Squamoid cyst of pancreatic ducts: a distinct type of cystic lesion in the pancreas. Am J Surg Pathol 2007;31:291–297.

31 Hanson JA, Salem RR, Mitchell KA: Squamoid cyst of pancreatic ducts: a case series describing novel immunohistochemistry, cytology, and quantitative cyst fluid chemistry. Arch Pathol Lab Med 2014;138:270–273.

32 Adsay NV, Hasteh F, Cheng JD, Bejarano PA, Lauwers GY, Batts KP, Kloppel G, Klimstra DS: Lymphoepithelial cysts of the pancreas: a report of 12 cases and a review of the literature. Mod Pathol 2002;15:492–501.

33 Ahlawat SK: Lymphoepithelial cyst of pancreas. Role of endoscopic ultrasound guided fine needle aspiration. JOP 2008;9:230–234.

34 Raval JS, Zeh HJ, Moser AJ, Lee KK, Sanders MK, Navina S, Kuan SF, Krasinskas AM: Pancreatic lymphoepithelial cysts express CEA and can contain mucous cells: potential pitfalls in the preoperative diagnosis. Mod Pathol 2010;23:1467–1476.

35 Dua KS, Vijayapal AS, Kengis J, Shidham VB: Ciliated foregut cyst of the pancreas: preoperative diagnosis using endoscopic ultrasound guided fine needle aspiration cytology – a case report with a review of the literature. Cytojournal 2009;6: 22.

36 Bellevicine C, Vigliar E, Pisapia P, de Luca C, Mazzarella C, Napolitano V, Troncone G: Ciliated foregut cyst of the pancreas: a benign lesion with elevated CEA levels. Diagn Cytopathol 2015;43: 178–180.

37 Weitman E, Al Diffalha S, Centeno B, Hodul P: An isolated intestinal duplication cyst masquerading as a mucinous cystic neoplasm of the pancreas: a case report and review of the literature. Int J Surg Case Rep 2017;39:208–211.

38 Woon CS, Pambuccian SE, Lai R, Jessurun J, Gulbahce HE: Ciliated foregut cyst of pancreas: cytologic findings on endoscopic ultrasound-guided fine-needle aspiration. Diagn Cytopathol 2007;35:433–438.

39 Huang H, Solanki MH, Giorgadze T: Cytomorphology of ciliated foregut cyst of the pancreas. Diagn Cytopathol 2019;47:347–350.

40 Alessandrino F, Allard FD, Mortele KJ: Ciliated pancreatic foregut cyst: MRI, EUS, and cytologic features. Clin Imaging 2016;40:140–143.

41 Jais B, Rebours V, Malleo G, Salvia R, Fontana M, Maggino L, et al: Serous cystic neoplasm of the pancreas: a multinational study of 2,622 patients under the auspices of the International Association of Pancreatology and European Pancreatic Club (European Study Group on Cystic Tumors of the Pancreas). Gut 2016;65:305–312.

42 Reid MD, Choi HJ, Memis B, Krasinskas AM, Jang KT, Akkas G, Maithel SK, Sarmiento JM, Kooby DA, Basturk O, Adsay V: Serous neoplasms of the pancreas: a clinicopathologic analysis of 193 cases and literature review with new insights on macrocystic and solid variants and critical reappraisal of so-called "serous cystadenocarcinoma." Am J Surg Pathol 2015;39:1597–1610.

43 Valsangkar NP, Morales-Oyarvide V, Thayer SP, Ferrone CR, Wargo JA, Warshaw AL, Fernandez-del Castillo C: 851 resected cystic tumors of the pancreas: a 33-year experience at the Massachusetts General Hospital. Surgery 2012;152(3 suppl 1):S4–S12.

44 Tseng JF, Warshaw AL, Sahani DV, Lauwers GY, Rattner DW, Fernandez-del Castillo C: Serous cystadenoma of the pancreas: tumor growth rates and recommendations for treatment. Ann Surg 2005;242:413–421.

45 Eras M, Yenigun M, Acar C, Kumbasar B, Sar F, Bilge T: Pancreatic involvement in von Hippel-Lindau disease. Indian J Cancer 2004;41:159–161.

46 Lewandrowski K, Lee J, Southern J, Centeno B, Warshaw A: Cyst fluid analysis in the differential diagnosis of pancreatic cysts: a new approach to the preoperative assessment of pancreatic cystic lesions. AJR Am J Roentgenol 1995;164:815–819.

47 Shah AA, Sainani NI, Kambadakone AR, Shah ZK, Deshpande V, Hahn PF, Sahani DV: Predictive value of multi-detector computed tomography for accurate diagnosis of serous cystadenoma: radiologic-pathologic correlation. World J Gastroenterol 2009;15:2739–2747.

48 Lewandrowski K, Warshaw A, Compton C: Macrocystic serous cystadenoma of the pancreas: a morphologic variant differing from microcystic adenoma. Hum Pathol 1992;23:871–875.

49 Kim SY, Lee JM, Kim SH, Shin KS, Kim YJ, An SK, Han CJ, Han JK, Choi BI: Macrocystic neoplasms of the pancreas: CT differentiation of serous oligocystic adenoma from mucinous cystadenoma and intraductal papillary mucinous tumor. AJR Am J Roentgenol 2006;187:1192–1198.

50 Machado MC, Machado MA: Solid serous adenoma of the pancreas: an uncommon but important entity. Eur J Surg Oncol 2008;34:730–733.

51 Kosmahl M, Wagner J, Peters K, Sipos B, Kloppel G: Serous cystic neoplasms of the pancreas: an immunohistochemical analysis revealing alpha-inhibin, neuron-specific enolase, and MUC6 as new markers. Am J Surg Pathol 2004;28:339–346.

52 Yamazaki K, Eyden B: An immunohistochemical and ultrastructural study of pancreatic microcystic serous cyst adenoma with special reference to tumor-associated microvasculature and vascular endothelial growth factor in tumor cells. Ultrastruct Pathol 2006;30:119–128.

53 Basturk O, Singh R, Kaygusuz E, Balci S, Dursun N, Culhaci N, Adsay NV: GLUT-1 expression in pancreatic neoplasia: implications in pathogenesis, diagnosis, and prognosis. Pancreas 2011;40:187–192.

54 Reid MD, Choi H, Balci S, Akkas G, Adsay V: Serous cystic neoplasms of the pancreas: clinicopathologic and molecular characteristics. Semin Diagn Pathol 2014;31:475–483.

55 Huang P, Staerkel G, Sneige N, Gong Y: Fine-needle aspiration of pancreatic serous cystadenoma: cytologic features and diagnostic pitfalls. Cancer 2006;108:239–249.

56 Collins BT: Serous cystadenoma of the pancreas with endoscopic ultrasound fine needle aspiration biopsy and surgical correlation. Acta Cytol 2013;57:241–251.

57 Belsley NA, Pitman MB, Lauwers GY, Brugge WR, Deshpande V: Serous cystadenoma of the pancreas: limitations and pitfalls of endoscopic ultrasound-guided fine-needle aspiration biopsy. Cancer 2008;114:102–110.

58 Jang KT, Park SM, Basturk O, Bagci P, Bandyopadhyay S, Stelow EB, Walters DM, Choi DW, Choi SH, Heo JS, Sarmiento JM, Reid MD, Adsay V: Clinicopathologic characteristics of 29 invasive carcinomas arising in 178 pancreatic mucinous cystic neoplasms with ovarian-type stroma: implications for management and prognosis. Am J Surg Pathol 2015;39:179–187.

59 Crippa S, Salvia R, Warshaw AL, Dominguez I, Bassi C, Falconi M, Thayer SP, Zamboni G, Lauwers GY, Mino-Kenudson M, Capelli P, Pederzoli P, Castillo CF: Mucinous cystic neoplasm of the pancreas is not an aggressive entity: lessons from 163 resected patients. Ann Surg 2008;247:571–579.

60 Farrell JJ: Prevalence, diagnosis and management of pancreatic cystic neoplasms: current status and future directions. Gut Liver 2015;9:571–589.

61 Griffin JF, Page AJ, Samaha GJ, Christopher A, Bhaijee F, Pezhouh MK, Peters NA, Hruban RH, He J, Makary MA, Lennon AM, Cameron JL, Wolfgang CL, Weiss MJ: Patients with a resected pancreatic mucinous cystic neoplasm have a better prognosis than patients with an intraductal papillary mucinous neoplasm: a large single institution series. Pancreatology 2017;17:490–496.

62 Tanaka M, Fernandez-Del Castillo C, Kamisawa T, Jang JY, Levy P, Ohtsuka T, Salvia R, Shimizu Y, Tada M, Wolfgang CL: Revisions of international consensus Fukuoka guidelines for the management of IPMN of the pancreas. Pancreatology 2017;17:738–753.

63 Genevay M, Mino-Kenudson M, Yaeger K, Konstantinidis IT, Ferrone CR, Thayer S, Castillo CF, Sahani D, Bounds B, Forcione D, Brugge WR, Pitman MB: Cytology adds value to imaging studies for risk assessment of malignancy in pancreatic mucinous cysts. Ann Surg 2011;254:977–983.

64 Basturk O, Hong SM, Wood LD, Adsay NV, Albores-Saavedra J, Biankin AV, Brosens LA, Fukushima N, Goggins M, Hruban RH, Kato Y, Klimstra DS, Kloppel G, Krasinskas A, Longnecker DS, Matthaei H, Offerhaus GJ, Shimizu M, Takaori K, Terris B, Yachida S, Esposito I, Furukawa T, Baltimore Consensus M: A revised classification system and recommendations from the baltimore consensus meeting for neoplastic precursor lesions in the pancreas. Am J Surg Pathol 2015;39:1730–1741.

65 Pitman MB, Centeno BA, Daglilar ES, Brugge WR, Mino-Kenudson M: Cytological criteria of high-grade epithelial atypia in the cyst fluid of pancreatic intraductal papillary mucinous neoplasms. Cancer Cytopathol 2014;122:40–47.

66 Basturk O, Tan M, Bhanot U, Allen P, Adsay V, Scott SN, Shah R, Berger MF, Askan G, Dikoglu E, Jobanputra V, Wrzeszczynski KO, Sigel C, Iacobuzio-Donahue C, Klimstra DS: The oncocytic subtype is genetically distinct from other pancreatic intraductal papillary mucinous neoplasm subtypes. Mod Pathol 2016;29:1058–1069.

67 La Rosa S, Sessa F, Capella C: Acinar cell carcinoma of the pancreas: overview of clinicopathologic features and insights into the molecular pathology. Front Med 2015;2:41.

68 Morales-Oyarvide V, Yoon WJ, Ingkakul T, Forcione DG, Casey BW, Brugge WR, Fernandez-del Castillo C, Pitman MB: Cystic pancreatic neuroendocrine tumors: the value of cytology in preoperative diagnosis. Cancer Cytopathol 2014;122:435–444.

69 Paal E, Thompson LD, Heffess CS: A clinicopathologic and immunohistochemical study of ten pancreatic lymphangiomas and a review of the literature. Cancer 1998;82:2150–2158.

70 Koenig TR, Loyer EM, Whitman GJ, Raymond AK, Charnsangavej C: Cystic lymphangioma of the pancreas. AJR Am J Roentgenol 2001;177:1090.

71 Casadei R, Minni F, Selva S, Marrano N, Marrano D: Cystic lymphangioma of the pancreas: anatomoclinical, diagnostic and therapeutic considerations regarding three personal observations and review of the literature. Hepatogastroenterology 2003;50:1681–1686.

72 Fonseca R, Pitman MB: Lymphangioma of the pancreas: a multimodal approach to pre-operative diagnosis. Cytopathology 2013;24:172–176.

73 Pitman MB, Centeno BA, Ali SZ, Genevay M, Stelow E, Mino-Kenudson M, et al: Standardized terminology and nomenclature for pancreatobiliary cytology: the Papanicolaou Society of Cytopathology guidelines. Diagn Cytopathol 2014;42:338–350.

Prof. Barbara A. Centeno
Department of Pathology, Moffitt Cancer Center
12902 USF Magnolia Drive
Tampa, FL 33612 (USA)
barbara.centeno@moffitt.org

Published online: September 29, 2020

Centeno BA, Dhillon J (eds): Pancreatic Tumors. Monogr Clin Cytol. Basel, Karger, 2020, vol 26, pp 74–91 (DOI:10.1159/000455736)

Pancreatic Ductal Adenocarcinoma

Jasreman Dhillon[a, b]   Michel Betancourt[c]

[a]Department of Anatomic Pathology, Moffitt Cancer Center, Tampa, FL, USA; [b]Department of Oncologic Sciences and Pathology, University of South Florida, Tampa, FL, USA; [c]Department of Pathology, Jupiter Medical Center, Jupiter, FL, USA

Abstract

The most frequent indication for pancreatic fine-needle aspiration sampling is to confirm or exclude a pancreatic ductal adenocarcinoma (PDAC). PDAC is the most common malignant neoplasm of the pancreas, and the term pancreatic cancer typically connotes this entity. The conventional type of PDAC is a tubular adenocarcinoma, with a number of morphological variations described. Morphologically distinct but related entities include adenosquamous carcinoma, undifferentiated carcinoma, and undifferentiated carcinoma with osteoclast-type giant cells. Unrelated carcinomas with ductal lineage include colloid carcinoma and medullary carcinoma. Less commonly reported carcinomas include signet ring cell carcinoma, hepatoid carcinoma, and oncocytic carcinoma. Here we will focus on the cytological findings of PDAC and other carcinomas of ductal lineage, briefly touching upon their clinical features, histologic appearance, and clinically useful serum markers. The differential diagnosis, pitfalls, and useful ancillary studies will also be reviewed. A diagnosis of PDAC should not be taken lightly given that it can potentially result in a pancreatic resection. Familiarity with the entities described in this review will help practicing cytopathologists confront these cases with appropriate information needed in order to render a clinically valuable diagnosis.   © 2020 S. Karger AG, Basel

Pancreatic ductal adenocarcinoma (PDAC) is the most common malignancy of the pancreas, accounting for 85–90% of all malignancies of the pancreas. Most often, patients are biopsied to confirm this disease. According to 2020 SEER data there will be estimated 57,600 new cases and 47,050 deaths of pancreatic carcinoma, which constitute 7.8% of all cancer deaths. Pancreatic cancer is a deadly disease with a 5-year relative survival rate of approximately 10%.

Clinical Presentation

PDAC and its variants (WHO 5th edition; Table 1) most typically occur in older adults, and most cases are diagnosed between the ages of 60 and 80 years. The most common tumor location is in the head of the pancreas (60–70%), consequently producing classic signs and symptoms of common bile duct obstruction and resultant hyperbilirubinemia such as jaundice, pruritus, dark urine, pale-colored stools, and a palpable gallbladder (Courvoisier's sign). Trousseau's sign (migratory thrombophlebitis) may be present in 10% of patients. It is useful to keep in mind that

Table 1. PDAC, variants, and individual types

Ductal carcinoma subtypes
WHO classification, 5th edition

Ductal adenocarcinoma
    Vacuolated pattern
    Foamy gland pattern
Adenosquamous carcinoma
Colloid carcinoma
Undifferentiated carcinoma, NOS
Undifferentiated carcinoma, anaplastic type
Undifferentiated carcinoma, sarcomatoid type
Undifferentiated carcinoma with osteoclast-like giant cells
Signet-ring cell carcinoma
Medullary carcinoma, NOS
Poorly cohesive carcinoma
Hepatoid carcinoma
Large-cell carcinoma with rhabdoid phenotype
Invasive micropapillary carcinoma

tumors arising in locations other than the head of the pancreas might not produce signs and symptoms related to common bile duct obstruction as described above. Other less specific symptoms include weight loss, malaise, nausea, fatigue, and mid-epigastric or back pain [1]. Patients can also present with cachexia, the severity of which does not correlate directly with tumor burden. Physical signs of distant metastasis include periumbilical metastasis (Sister Mary Joseph nodule) and left supraclavicular lymph node metastasis (Virchow's node). Abnormal laboratory values associated with PDAC may include elevated fasting glucose levels, hyperbilirubinemia, and elevated serum pancreatic enzymes [2, 3].

Serum markers in PDAC are primarily used for monitoring the disease progression and seldom for screening purposes as in patients with hereditary pancreatitis where the incidence of PDAC is higher than in the general population. Carbohydrate antigen 19-9 (CA19-9) is the most commonly used serum marker in the setting of pancreatic cancer. CA19-9 is the most useful blood test in differentiating pancreatic cancer from chronic and recurring pancreatitis, and is also the most significant prognostic factor for patients with PDAC [4]. An elevated CA19-9 value immediately after resection indicates a high possibility of remnant disease [5]. Changes in CA19-9 levels may help in evaluating the tumor response to chemotherapy and/or radiotherapy treatments. CA19-9 is a result of a molecular modification to the Lewis antigen; therefore, an important caveat to its use is that patients who are Lewis antigen negative (Le^{a-b-}) will not express CA19-9 (5–10% of the population). In these patients, serum levels of CA19-9 can be either normal or decreased despite a high tumor burden [6]. Carcinoembryonic antigen (CEA) is another serum marker commonly used in clinical practice to monitor PDAC. It suffers from a lower sensitivity than CA19-9 while its specificity is comparable [2]. It has largely been replaced by other markers for monitoring pancreatic cancer patients. CA125 is a high-molecular-weight glycoprotein and is expressed in ovarian cancer and pancreatic cancer cells. This marker can be more useful than CA19-9 in the setting of hyperbilirubinemia [3]. However, CA125 also suffers from lack of specificity and poor sensitivity. Other serum markers which have been proposed but are not yet in clinical use are CA242, TPA, TPS, M2-pyruvate kinase, Mic-1, IGFBP-1a, Du-Pan, haptoglobin, and serum amyloid A [7].

Imaging Studies

The imaging findings of PDAC and utilization of imaging for staging are covered in the chapter by Morse and Klapman [this vol., pp. 21–33]. Endoscopic ultrasound (EUS) characteristics of PDAC are the presence of a hypoechoic mass and double duct sign. The most common cause of double duct sign is pancreatic adenocarcinoma. Typical findings on computed tomography (CT) scans include a poorly defined mass that appears hypodense in the majority of cases and is surrounded by an area suggestive of desmoplastic reaction. A double duct sign may be present. Other signs that can be observed with a CT scan are extension of the tumor beyond the pancreatic parenchyma, pancreatic enlargement, and dilatation and/or obstruction of the pancreatic duct or common bile duct. EUS imaging may also show a double duct sign and extension beyond the pancreas.

Ductal Adenocarcinoma, Conventional Type
Histology
The histological appearance of conventional PDAC is characterized by the formation of neoplastic, mucin-producing glands that infiltrate into the adjoining tissue, accompanied by a dense, desmoplastic stromal reaction. Malignant glands infiltrate in a disorganized and haphazard fashion, with loss of normal pancreatic lobular architecture (Fig. 1a). Malignant glands adjacent to a muscularized vessel are evidence of PDAC, as are perineural and lymphovascular invasion. The nuclei are enlarged and vary in size and shape. Anisonucleosis of >4:1 is a diagnostic feature. As the PDAC be-

comes less differentiated, gland formation and cytoplasmic mucin production decrease, and mitotic activity and nuclear atypia increase. The cytoplasm may vary from eosinophilic to clear or foamy, and these cytoplasmic patterns may be seen on histology (Fig. 1b). Perineural and angiolymphatic invasion are evidence of PDAC either in a core biopsy or cell block sections containing intact stromal fragments.

Cytology

A cytological diagnosis of conventional PDAC rests on assessing the cellularity, cellular composition, background, architectural pattern, nuclear features, and cytoplasmic contents. Malignant processes are typically more cellular than benign or reactive processes, but paucicellular samples can occur in PDAC as a result of extensive desmoplasia. The background of aspirates from PDAC may be clean, bloody, necrotic, mucinous, or inflammatory (Fig. 1c) as compared to benign aspirates which are usually clean or at times inflammatory. Malignant ductal groups lose their normal honeycomb pattern and demonstrate crowding and overlapping of nuclei (Fig. 1d), or else an exaggerated honeycomb pattern due to an excess of cytoplasmic mucin (Fig. 1e). Cellular dyshesion is a feature of malignancy, and single cells with nuclear features of malignancy are diagnostic of PDAC (Fig. 1f). Pseudoacinar formations and cribriforming may occur (Fig. 1g). These architectural abnormalities may be discernible at low to intermediate power. Nuclear features assessed include the nuclear size, nuclear-to-cytoplasmic ratio, nuclear shape, and chromatin pattern. Malignant nuclei are larger, measuring at least 1.5 times the

size of a red blood cell on a Diff-Quik smear. Typically, the nuclear-to-cytoplasmic ratio is increased in PDAC, except in cases with abundant cytoplasmic mucin, in which the overall size of the cell is increased. The nuclei lose their round, smooth shape and become elongated, with pointed edges, nuclear infoldings, or grooves (Fig. 1h). More atypical cells will show nuclear membrane convolutions. Anisonucleosis in a ratio of >4:1 is a feature of malignancy (Fig. 1i). The chromatin pattern in PDAC may be hypochromatic or hyperchromatic. An irregular parachromatin clearing may be identified. Normal ductal cells do not contain cytoplasmic mucin, so the presence of cytoplasmic mucin in ductal-type epithelium in the pancreas is abnormal. Cells may be elongated and columnar, vacuolated, or else have a single prominent mucin vacuole (Fig. 1j). Both reactive and malignant processes may exhibit mitotic figures, but abnormal mitotic figures are a feature of malignancy. Prominent nucleoli are not a specific feature. These features described are qualitative [8–11]. A few studies have published the minimum number of criteria that are needed for a diagnosis of PDAC [11]. Quantitative criteria have not been established for the diagnosis of malignancy. However, one retrospective study reported that all of the malignant aspirates in their study had at least 6 groups with a combination of the criteria listed above. The differences between a benign pancreatic aspirate and a malignant pancreatic aspirate are listed in Table 2 (Fig. 1k).

The characteristic appearance of PDAC is an adenocarcinoma with cuboidal cells, a finely vacuolated cytoplasm, and raisinoid nuclei, appreciated on cell block sections. This morphology is the correlate of the exaggerated honeycomb

Fig. 1. Morphological features of PDAC. **a** Malignant cells forming glands that are infiltrating in a haphazard manner. HE stain, ×10. **b** Histological section showing tumor cells with eosinophilic to clear and vacuolated cytoplasm. HE stain, ×40. **bi–iii** Cytological features of PDAC with a vacuolated cell pattern. **bi** Cluster of tumor cells exhibiting features of malignancy with a large intracytoplasmic vacuole in one of them. Diff-Quik stain, ×60. **bii** Malignant tumor cells, many of which have large intracytoplasmic vacuoles. Papanicolaou stain, ×60. **biii** Cell block section showing infiltrating tumor cells exhibiting a vacuolated cytoplasm. HE stain, ×40. **c** Tumor cells admixed with acute inflammatory cells. Diff-Quik stain, ×40. **ci** Foamy gland pattern. Tumor cells with basally located nuclei, microvesicular cytoplasm, and a brush border-like luminal zone. HE stain, ×20. **d** Tumor cells with crowded and overlapping nuclei. Diff-Quik stain, ×40. **e** Tumor cells with intracytoplasmic mucin giving an exaggerated honeycomb pattern. Papanicolaou stain, ×40. **f** Tumor cells present in loose aggregates and as single cells. Diff-Quik stain, ×20. **g** Tumor cells with cribriforming present in a cell block section. HE stain, ×40. **h** Tumor cells with pleomorphic nuclei exhibiting nuclear grooves and irregular and pointed ends. Papanicolaou stain, ×40. **i** Tumor cells with >4:1 anisonucleosis. Papanicolaou stain, ×40. **j** Tumor cells with mucinous cytoplasm. Diff-Quik, ×60. **k** A cluster of tumor cells (center) with two adjacent clusters of benign duodenal epithelial cells. Papanicolaou stain, ×20. **l** A cellular cluster of well-differentiated PDAC with a clean background. Diff-Quik stain, ×20. **m** Loss of polarity and anisonucleosis in a well-differentiated PDAC. Papanicolaou stain, ×40. **n** Well-differentiated PDAC with a "drunken" honeycomb appearance. Papanicolaou stain, ×60. **o** Well-differentiated PDAC showing subtle variation in nuclear size in a ratio of >4:1 in the lower aspect of the image. Papanicolaou stain, ×60. **p** Well-differentiated PDAC with variation in nuclear size and shape. Diff-Quik stain, ×60. **q** Poorly differentiated PDAC with markedly pleomorphic tumor cells with nuclear overlapping and loss of honeycomb pattern. Diff-Quik stain, ×40. **r** Poorly differentiated group of PDAC with a mitotic figure. Papanicolaou stain, ×60.

(For figure see next pages.)

appearance seen on smears. When identified at distant sites, it is highly suggestive of a pancreatic primary. Grading of PDAC is not typically performed on fine-needle aspiration biopsy (FNAB), but it is worth noting that the qualitative criteria described above are subtler in well-differentiated PDAC compared to a higher-grade PDAC [9]. One of the studies showed that the cytologic grade of pancreatic adeno-carcinoma independently predicted survival in these pa-tients [12]. Cytologic features associated with worse surviv-al in this study were the presence of necrosis, bizarre cells, 3-dimensional dyscohesive groups, many single tumor cells, and the absence of mucin. FNAB of a well-differentiated

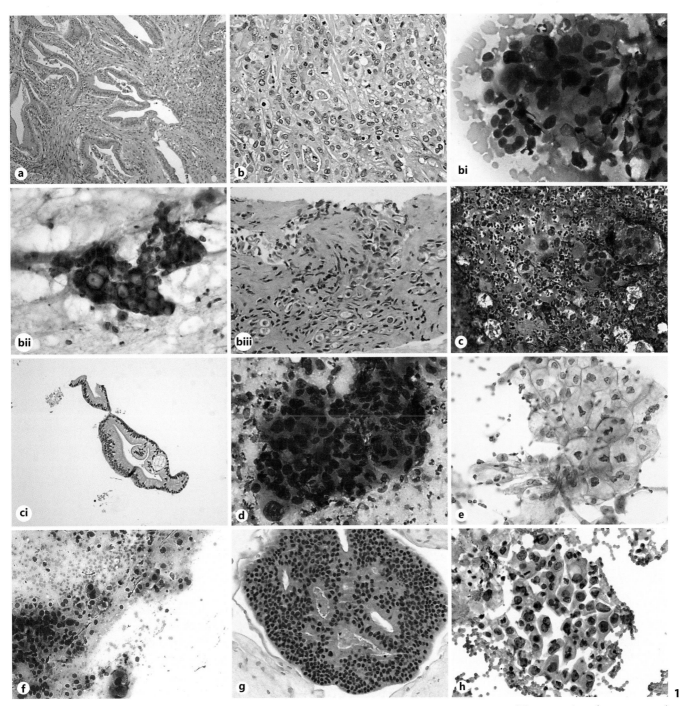

(Figure continued on next page.)

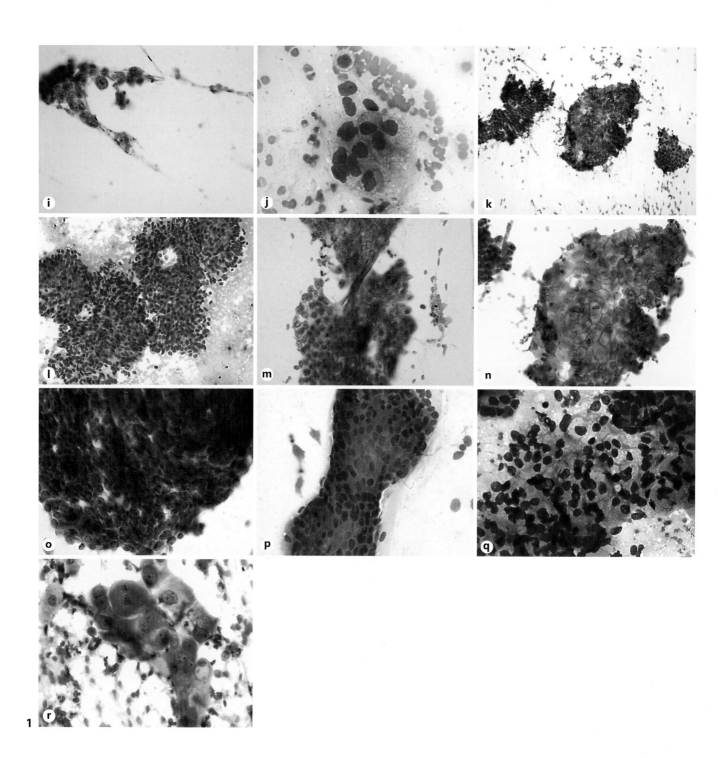

PDAC frequently results in highly cellular smears with a clean background (Fig. 1l), showing sheets of cohesive ductal cells with nuclear crowding and loss of nuclear polarity or a "drunken" or exaggerated honeycomb appearance (Fig. 1m, n). Nuclear changes include anisonucleosis of 4:1, an irregular chromatin distribution, and nuclear membrane irregularities (Fig. 1o, p) [1]. Single tumor cells are few to absent and the cytoplasm can contain mucin vacuoles [2, 3]. Table 3 illustrates the cytological differences between a well-differentiated PDAC and a moderately or poorly differentiated PDAC.

Table 2. Differences between pancreatic adenocarcinoma and benign pancreatic aspirates

Cytological feature assessed	Benign pancreatic aspirate	Malignant pancreatic aspirate
Cellularity	Less	Increased
Background	Clean or dirty/necrotic and inflammatory in pancreatitis	Bloody, necrotic, mucinous, inflammatory
Cellular clusters	One-dimensional clusters with honeycombing	Three-dimensional, loosely cohesive clusters with loss of polarity
Single cells	Usually absent	Present
Nuclear size	Small	Larger than normal (1.5× RBC)
Nuclear/cytoplasmic ratio	Not increased	Increased except in mucinous carcinoma, PDAC with vacuolated cell pattern and foamy gland pattern
Nuclear shape	Round with smooth nuclear contour	Oval with irregular nuclear contour
Anisonucleosis	Absent to minimal	Present in a ratio of 4:1 or more
Chromatin pattern	Isochromatic without coarse chromatin clumping	Hypochromatic, hyperchromatic, coarse chromatin clumping present
Cytoplasmic mucin	Absent in pancreatic epithelial cells	Present
Mitotic figures	Normal mitotic spindle, if present	Atypical mitotic figures present

Table 3. Differences between a well-differentiated pancreatic adenocarcinoma and a high-grade (moderately and poorly) differentiated adenocarcinoma

Cytological criteria assessed	Well-differentiated adenocarcinoma	Poorly differentiated adenocarcinoma
Background	Clean	Dirty, necrotic
Architecture	Cohesive	Dyshesion evident, single cells
Nuclear membrane irregularities	Subtle, angulated	Nuclear convolutions
Chromatin	Hypochromasia more common	Hyperchormasia more common
Anisonucleosis	Mild	Marked

Smears from moderately and poorly differentiated PDAC can reveal highly cellular samples with a necrotic or inflammatory background. The cells lose their cytoplasmic differentiation. Degrees of anisocytosis and nuclear membrane irregularities are more pronounced in moderate to poorly differentiated PDAC than in well-differentiated tumors (Fig. 1q). In addition, single cells and atypical mitotic figures are more readily identified in poorly differentiated PDAC (Fig. 1r).

Key Cytological Features
   Well-differentiated PDAC:
- Clean background
- Cohesive sheets of ductal cells with crowded nuclei and variable N/C ratios
- Anisonucleosis
- Hypochromasia
- Subtler nuclear atypia characterized by elongated, pointy, or angulated nuclei
   Moderately to poorly differentiated PDAC:
- Background necrosis more common

- Groups with nuclear crowding and overlapping, or an exaggerated honeycomb
- Marked anisonucleosis
- Nuclear membrane irregularities with readily evident nuclear convolutions
- Hyperchromasia, hypochromasia, and irregular parachromatin clearing
- Atypical mitotic figures
- Single malignant cells

Ancillary Studies

PDAC has a non-specific immunoprofile where the tumor cells generally stain for CK7, CK8, CK18, CK19, and BAP1. Over the past few years, many tissue-based markers, such as K-ras, p53, specific mucins (MUC1, 2, 4, 5AC), p21, BCl-2, SMAD4, and microRNAs, have been described which can be helpful in establishing a diagnosis of PDAC [6]. *K-ras* is one of the most frequently mutated oncogenes which are responsible for signals resulting in increased cell proliferation, enhanced cell survival, and resistance to apoptosis. Approximately 90% of PDAC cases are *K-ras* mutated. The *p53* tumor-suppressor gene regulates the expression of genes involved in apoptosis, angiogenesis, and the cell cycle, and is found altered in 50–70% of pancreatic cancers [13]. Mucins, especially MUC1 and MUC5AC, are overexpressed in PDAC. Wang et al. [14] showed that combining MUC1 and MUC5AC with cytology yielded higher sensitivity and specificity in diagnosing PDAC. A panel of MUC1+, MUC2−, and MUC5AC+ was more specific for a diagnosis of PDAC. Similarly, MUC4 is also useful in establishing a diagnosis of PDAC. *SMAD4*, also known as *DPC4*, is a tumor-suppressor gene that is inactivated in a subset of PDAC. Absence of immunohistochemical staining for SMAD4/DPC4 proteins can be used as an important marker for confirming the diagnosis of pancreatic adenocarcinoma, and for confirming the site of origin as the pancreas [15]. It has been shown that patients undergoing surgical resection for pancreatic adenocarcinoma survive longer if their cancers express SMAD4 [16]. Insulin-like growth factor II messenger ribonucleic acid-binding protein 3 (IMP3) is a marker for malignancy which correlates with increased tumor aggressiveness and reduced overall survival [17]. PDAC usually exhibits a strong staining pattern with IMP3, whereas benign pancreatic tissue either does not stain or stains weakly.

Differential Diagnosis

There is a broad differential diagnosis that can range from benign, inflammatory processes to other malignant tumors in the pancreas. It is usually difficult to distinguish a well-differentiated PDAC from benign, reactive, and inflammatory processes. Aspirates of the normal pancreas are composed of acinar cells and rarely islet cells, which can be seen in pancreatic atrophy. Acinar cells are arranged in small acinar-shaped structures and have a moderate to abundant amount of granular cytoplasm. It is important to recognize these cells as normal components of the pancreas and not to overinterpret them to be neoplastic. The normal ductal epithelium is columnar or cuboidal and is present as flat, honeycombed, 2-dimensional sheets. The nuclei are either centrally located or palisaded. It is important to distinguish mucinous epithelial contaminants from gastric, and duodenal epithelium from PDAC. Benign epithelium is typically monolayered, usually with a luminal border at one edge of the aggregate. In comparison, tumor aspirates are usually crowded, hypercellular groups of cells with cribriforming and loss of nuclear polarity. Nuclear abnormalities as described above are present and will be helpful in reaching the correct diagnosis [18].

Aspirates from inflammatory processes, such as acute and chronic pancreatitis, autoimmune pancreatitis, and lymphoplasmacytic pancreatitis, are usually dirty with a necrotic background and cellular debris. A variable number of inflammatory cells may be present. The pancreatic ductal epithelium shows reactive atypia such as nuclear enlargement, subtle anisonucleosis, coarse chromatin, and prominent nucleoli [19]. It is important not to overinterpret these findings. Other sources of reactive atypia include the radiation effect and stents. Pancreatic intraepithelial neoplasia is reported to be one of the sources of pitfalls in diagnosis [19]. Cytomorphological findings must be correlated with the clinical history, imaging findings, and presentation to make a correct diagnosis and avoid pitfalls.

Morphological Patterns or Variations of PDAC, Conventional Type

A few histomorphological patterns have been described, including the large duct pattern, vacuolated cell pattern, and foamy gland pattern. Herein, we describe the patterns that can be recognized on cytology, the vacuolated cell pattern, and the foamy gland pattern (Table 4).

PDAC with Vacuolated Cell Pattern
Histology

This tumor is a morphologic variant of PDAC and not a separate entity. The clinical presentation is similar to PDAC. This neoplasm is characterized by infiltrating nests of tumor cells with large vacuoles imparting a cribriform growth pat-

Table 4. Summary of PDACs with immunophenotypic and molecular features

Ductal carcinoma type	Key cytological features	Immunohistochemistry and molecular alterations
Ductal adenocarcinoma, conventional type	Gland-forming tumor with malignant cytological features	Pan-CK, CK7, CK8/18, CK19/MUC1, MUC5AC Mutations involve *KRAS*, *TP53*, *DPC4* genes
Vacuolated cell	Tumor cells with large intracytoplasmic vacuoles No background mucin	CK7, CK8/18, CA19-9, MUC1, 34βE12 Intracytoplasmic vacuoles stain positive for mucicarmine and PAS-AB Mutations involve *KRAS* gene
Foamy gland	Tumor cells with a foamy cytoplasm and a low N/C ratio Basally located nuclei with brush border-like zone	CK8, CEA, MUC1 Mutations involving *KRAS* and *TP53* genes
Adenosquamous carcinoma	Mixed glandular and squamous malignant components	As above and squamous markers CK5/6, p63, and p40 Mutations involve *KRAS* and *DPC4* genes
Undifferentiated (anaplastic) carcinoma	Mononucleated, pleomorphic cells Pleomorphic, multinucleated cells	CK, vimentin, loss of membranous β-catenin and E-cadherin
Rhabdoid type	Pleomorphic tumor cells with predominant (>50%) rhabdoid cells Monomorphic tumor cells with predominant (>50%) rhabdoid cells	CK, vimentin Pleomorphic subtype with *KRAS* mutations and intact INI1 (SMARCB1) Monomorphic subtype with loss of INI1 (SMARCB1), *KRAS* intact
Undifferentiated carcinoma with osteoclast-like giant cells	Mononucleated, pleomorphic cells Osteoclast-type benign multinucleated cells	CK focally present, vimentin+ Osteoclasts – LCA, vimentin, CD68, KP1
Colloid (mucinous non-cystic) carcinoma	Background mucin with malignant glands	MUC1, MUC2, CDX 2+
SRCC	Signet ring cells floating in pools of mucin	CKs, 7, 8/18, 19, CEA, MUC1, MUC5AC
Medullary carcinoma	Syncytial groups of malignant cells Lymphocytic infiltrate	Few with loss of MMR proteins, Mutations involving *KRAS* and *BRAF* genes
Hepatoid carcinoma	Tumor cells with round nuclei and abundant eosinophilic, granular cytoplasm	HepPAR1, AFP
Oncocytic carcinoma	Oncocytic tumor cells with round nuclei, prominent nucleoli Nuclear grooves and pseudoinclusions present	MUC1, MUC6 and anti-mitochondrial antibody 113-1 No mutations involving *KRAS* and *TP53* genes

CK, cytokeratin; MMR, mismatch repair proteins; AFP, alpha fetoprotein; SRCC, signet ring cell carcinoma; PAS-AB, periodic acid Schiff-Alcian blue.

tern [20, 21]. The intracytoplasmic vacuoles are 1–5 times the cell size. Merger of these vacuolated cells forms a multilocular space which is separated by a thin rim of cell membrane. These spaces may contain cellular debris and mucin. The nuclei are compressed and pushed to the periphery, resembling adipocytes [21]. The nuclei are pleomorphic, hyperchromatic, and enlarged.

Cytology

FNA smears show the tumor cells that are predominantly present in aggregates, and few as single cells. There is background necrotic debris but no background mucin. Individual cells have a low nuclear-to-cytoplasmic ratio and vacuolated cytoplasm [22]. The cytoplasm is metachromatic with internal granularity. Although the tumor cells have a low nucleus-to-cytoplasmic ratio, presence of other cytologic features of malignancy, such as nuclear overlapping, loss of cohesiveness, loss of honeycomb architecture, anisonucleosis (>4:1), irregular nuclear contours, prominent nucleoli, and atypical chromatin, are helpful in establishing a diagnosis of malignancy (Fig. 1.bi–iii). The tumor cells may have a squamoid appearance, but no definite features of squamous differentiation, such as keratinization or intercellular bridges, are present.

Key Cytological Features
• Necrotic debris may be present in the background
• Tumor cells present predominantly in aggregates
• Individual tumor cells have a low N/C ratio
• There is a very large intracytoplasmic vacuole occupying most of the cytoplasm
• Nucleus is pushed to the periphery
• Nucleus is hyperchromatic and pleomorphic
• There is no background mucin

Ancillary Studies
Vacuolated tumor cells that contain mucin stain positive for mucicarmine and PAS-Alcian blue. The tumor cells generally stain as PDAC stains. They stain for CA19-9, MUC1, and CEA. However, unlike PDAC, many stain positive for high molecular cytokeratin 34βE12. Most of the tumors are *KRAS* mutated and have the same molecular alterations as conventional PDAC.

Differential Diagnosis
The large vacuolated cells may resemble degenerating adipocytes present in fat necrosis, lipogranulomas present in lymph nodes, and may resemble lipoblasts in liposarcoma [21]. Primary pancreatic signet ring cell carcinoma (SRCC) or metastatic SRCCs to the pancreas must be distinguished from this variant. In SRCCs, tumor cells are dyscohesive and infiltrate individually as single cells. Signet ring cells are present as single cells in mucin pools and are negative for E-cadherin and β-catenin. They have relatively smaller vacuoles with less nuclear atypia, whereas the tumor cells in the vacuolated variant of pancreatic cancer are predominantly present as cellular aggregates without background mucin.

PDAC with Foamy Gland Pattern (or Foamy Gland Adenocarcinoma)
Histology
Foamy gland adenocarcinoma of the pancreas is a deceptively benign-appearing variant of PDAC which is charac-

terized by a prominent microvesicular cytoplasm giving tumor cells a foamy appearance [23]. The nuclei in the tumor cells are often basally located, compressed, and hyperchromatic (Fig. 1ci). Some of the nuclei have irregular nuclear membranes imparting a raisinoid appearance. There is condensation of cytoplasmic material in the luminal aspect of the tumor cells that imparts a brush border-like zone that stains positive for mucicarmine and Alcian blue but is negative for PAS [23].

Cytology
The smears may show tumor cells that are predominantly composed of a foamy gland pattern or an admixture of foamy gland pattern with typical PDAC cells. The tumor cells exhibit a low nuclear-to-cytoplasmic ratio, foamy cytoplasm, and loss of honeycomb architecture. The tumor cells may exhibit well demarcated cell borders, clumpy chromatin with prominent nucleoli, and irregular nuclear contours [20]. Almost all the cases exhibit cytological features of conventional PDAC in addition to the foamy tumor cells.

Key Cytological Findings
• Tumor cells with a low nuclear-to-cytoplasmic ratio
• Foamy cytoplasm
• Basally located nuclei with cribriforming
• Admixed conventional PDAC

Ancillary Studies
The brush border-like zone in the tumor cells stains positive for mucicarmine and Alcian blue and negative for PAS. The tumor cells stain positive for CEA, CK8, and focally for B72.3. MUC1 staining is confined to the brush border-like zone. MUC2 is negative. The neoplastic cells may have *KRAS* mutations and express p53.

Differential Diagnosis
This tumor may be mistaken for benign mucinous ductal epithelial cells and either misdiagnosed as benign or understaged. However, attention to subtle morphologic features such as the presence of raisinoid, hyperchromatic nuclei, and presence of a brush border-like zone are useful in recognizing the cells as malignant. PAS stain can be helpful in distinguishing the two as benign mucinous cells stain positive whereas the tumor cells do not stain with PAS.

Related Carcinomas
We will now briefly discuss the other distinct entities of ductal lineage occurring in the pancreas (Table 3), providing an

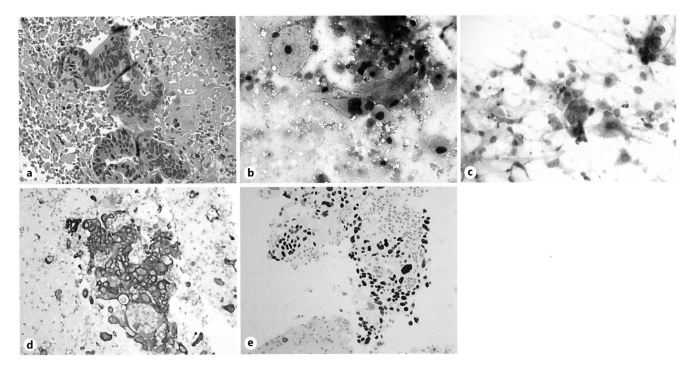

Fig. 2. Adenosquamous carcinoma. **a** Cell block section with an adenocarcinoma component in the middle and squamous cell carcinoma component present adjacent to it admixed with necrosis. HE stain, ×40. **b** Tumor cells with squamous differentiation present in the form of a tadpole cell and dense cytoplasm. Diff-Quik stain, ×60. **c** Tumor cells with an adenocarcinoma component and squamous carcinoma component with characteristic orangeophilia. Papanicolaou stain, ×60. **d** Squamous cell carcinoma component staining for immunostain CK5/6, ×20. **e** Squamous cell carcinoma component staining for immunostain p40, ×20.

overview of their histology, cytology, ancillary studies, and differential diagnosis.

Adenosquamous Carcinoma

Histology

This is the most common variant of PDAC. Histological and cytological appearances are both characterized by a mixture of squamous and glandular malignant epithelial proliferation (Fig. 2a). Various theories proposed for histogenesis of adenosquamous carcinoma are squamous metaplasia resulting from ductal inflammation or obstruction; these are two different tumors that arise independently and join together and the differentiation theory which states that a primitive pancreatic stem cell differentiates into squamous and adenocarcinoma and becomes a combination of both [24, 25]. According to the WHO classification, the lesser component should represent at least 30% of the tumor. Although this cut-off is arbitrary, an even lesser amount of squamous differentiation can portend a worse prognosis. The percentage of the squamous component cannot be determined accurately on FANB.

Given that primary squamous cell carcinoma of the pancreas is essentially non-existent, any malignant squamous epithelium might prompt suspicion of this variant. This is of importance because adenosquamous carcinoma has a poorer prognosis when compared to conventional PDAC [1]. The malignant squamous component may predominate or it may be scant, and it may be either keratinizing or non-keratinizing [2].

Cytology

Smears show clusters of malignant epithelial cells with glandular and squamous differentiation although one component may predominate and the other may be focal. Squamous differentiation may be appreciated on smears by the presence of tadpole cells, clusters of tumor cells with intercellular junctions and dense cytoplasm, and characteristic orangeophilia on Papanicolaou-stained slides (Fig. 2b, c). The background may be necrotic with the presence of keratinous debris. Malignant glandular epithelial cells with intracellular mucin are present [26].

Key Cytological Features
- Necrosis, often including keratinized debris
- Malignant keratinized or non-keratinized squamous cells
- Tadpole cells may be present
- Characteristic orangeophilia on Papanicolaou-stained smears
- Adenocarcinoma component

Ancillary Studies

The glandular component of the tumor stains positive for CK7 and the squamous component stains positive for CK5/6, p40, and p63 (Fig. 2d, e). Intracellular mucin can be highlighted in the glandular cells by special stains for mucin, such as mucicarmine. The tumor focally stains positive for CK20 and stains negative for p16 and p53. CA19-9 stains both components. This carcinoma has similar mutations to conventional PDAC, including KRAS mutations and loss of DPC4 [27].

Differential Diagnosis

Adenosquamous carcinoma of the pancreas must be distinguished from a pure adenocarcinoma of the pancreas with accompanying squamous metaplasia of the pancreatic ducts. Metastatic squamous cell carcinomas to the pancreas from other organs must be distinguished from a primary adenosquamous carcinoma, where the squamous component is predominant, as primary squamous cell carcinomas of the pancreas are very rare.

Undifferentiated (Anaplastic) Carcinoma
Histology

This variant of PDAC has an extremely poor prognosis and is more aggressive with a median survival of 5.2 months as patients typically present with widely metastatic disease. The tumor has a male predominance [28]. The tumor is typically of a soft consistency due to a lack of desmoplasia compared to conventional PDAC. The histological appearance is varied; however, it is typically a tumor of pleomorphic cells with the occurrence of pleomorphic multinucleated cells. Components of conventional PDAC, squamous differentiation, spindle cells, and heterologous elements can be present. This variant can be associated with a substantial acute inflammatory background (Fig. 3a).

Cytology

FANB smears are very cellular with large, cohesive tissue fragments with dispersed large and bizarre single cells. The malignant cells can be mononuclear or multinucleated and can occasionally have a sarcomatoid, spindled appearance [29]. Other findings include frequent mitotic figures, marked inflammation, and phagocytosis of inflammatory cells and red blood cells by tumoral cells (Fig. 3b). This tumor is known to coexpress cytokeratin and vimentin, a finding that can be useful if the available cell block material is appropriate for ancillary studies [30]. Recently, two variants of undifferentiated carcinoma have been described which are associated with a predominant rhabdoid morphology [31]. These are pleomorphic type with rhabdoid cells and monomorphic type with rhabdoid cells (Fig. 3c).

Key Cytological Features
- Highly cellular smears
- Pleomorphic multinucleated giant cells
- Oval to spindle cells
- Background necrosis and inflammation
- Presence of mitotic figures
- Cytophagocytosis
- Rhabdoid cells in rhabdoid variants

Ancillary Studies

The tumor cells generally coexpress cytokeratins and vimentin (Fig. 3d). Immunohistochemistry for p53 is usually positive, correlating with mutation in this gene. There is typically loss of E-cadherin (Fig. 3e). Loss of INI1 (SMARCB1) expression has been reported in the rhabdoid variant, especially the monomorphic subtype (Fig. 3f) [31]. The pleomorphic subtype is usually reported to have an intact INI1 expression with mutations in the KRAS gene [31].

Differential Diagnosis

This tumor should be differentiated from undifferentiated carcinoma with osteoclast-like giant cells as the latter has a better prognosis. Both entities have spindle cells with the presence of giant cells. However, the giant cells present in undifferentiated carcinoma are pleomorphic and those present in undifferentiated carcinoma with osteoclast-like giant cells are non-neoplastic osteoclast-like giant cells with a characteristic staining pattern as described below.

Undifferentiated Carcinoma with Osteoclast-Like Giant Cells
Histology

Many names have been given to this variant, such as giant cell tumor of the pancreas and osteoclastoma, among others. The clinical presentation is similar to that of conven-

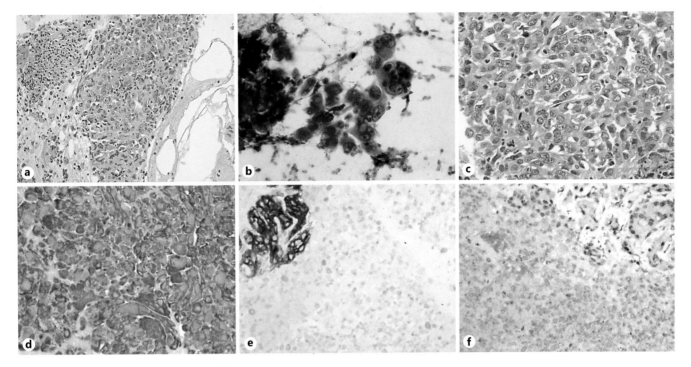

Fig. 3. Undifferentiated carcinoma. **a** Pleomorphic tumor cells admixed with acute inflammatory cells. HE stain, ×20. **b** Pleomorphic tumor cells phagocytosing inflammatory cells. Papanicolaou stain, ×40. **c** Undifferentiated carcinoma with rhabdoid cells, ×40. **d** Tumor cells staining positive for immunostain vimentin, ×40. **e** Tumor cells with loss of E-cadherin immunostain. Normal ductal epithelial cells with retention of the staining, ×40. **f** Tumor cells with loss of INI-1 and normal expression in the benign acinar cells, ×40.

tional PDAC. The mean age of presentation is 60 years. Histological features include the presence of both mononuclear tumor cells with significant nuclear pleomorphism, and non-neoplastic osteoclast-like giant cells (Fig. 4a). The osteoclast-like giant cells are multinucleated cells with the presence of usually >20 round and uniform nuclei. Osteoclast-like giant cells are more noticeable around areas of necrosis and hemorrhage. This variant can have osteoid or chondroid differentiation.

Cytology
FNAB smears show a dual population of pleomorphic mononuclear cells and multinucleated osteoclast-like giant cells with bland-appearing, centrally located nuclei (Fig. 4b, c). Sarcomatoid cells and abnormal mitotic figures can also be present [32, 33].

Key Cytological Features
- Large tissue fragments and single cells
- Pleomorphic mononuclear epithelial cells
- Osteoclast-like giant cells
- Sarcomatoid cells
- Abnormal mitotic figures

Ancillary Studies
The ductal carcinoma foci stain positive for cytokeratins and CAM5.2. Pleomorphic spindle cells (sarcomatoid component) stain positive for vimentin. The osteoclast-like giant cells stain positive for leucocyte common antigen, vimentin, and macrophage markers such as CD68, KP1, and stain negative for cytokeratins and p53 (Fig. 4d, e).

Differential Diagnosis
This tumor should be differentiated from undifferentiated carcinoma.

Colloid (Mucinous Non-Cystic) Carcinoma
Histology
This variant differs from conventional-type PDAC in that it is well circumscribed in radiologic studies and on gross examination, with occasional calcifications. There may be a slight male prediction in colloid carcinoma [34]. Colloid

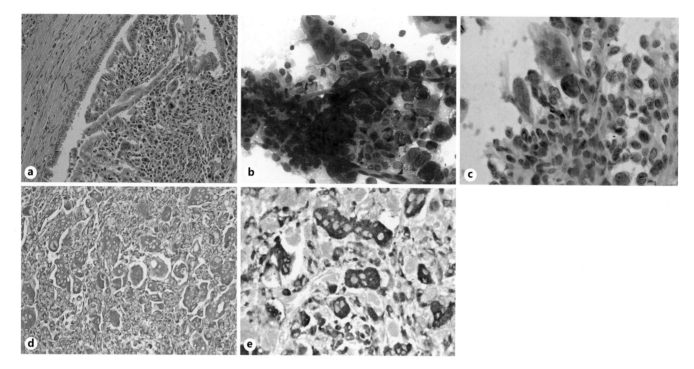

Fig. 4. Undifferentiated carcinoma with osteoclast-like giant cells. **a** Tumor cells with admixed non-neoplastic osteoclast-like giant cells involving a benign pancreatic duct. HE stain, ×20. **b** A sheet of pleomorphic tumor cells and osteoclast-like giant cells. Diff-Quik stain, ×40. **c** Pleomorphic tumor cell nuclei as compared to the benign nuclei of the osteoclast-like giant cell. Papanicolaou stain, ×60. **d** The tumor cells as well as the osteoclast-like giant cells staining positive for immunostain vimentin, ×20. **e** Osteoclast-like multinucleated cells staining positive for immunostain CD68, ×40.

carcinoma has a significantly improved long-term survival compared to typical PDAC. These arise exclusively in association with intestinal-type intraductal papillary mucinous neoplasms (IPMNs). Histologically, this variant is characterized by pools of mucin, accounting for at least 80% of the tumor (Fig. 5a). Mucin is associated with cuboidal adenocarcinoma cells either singly or forming strips of malignant epithelium. The tumor cells are present floating in pools of stromal mucin. This variant is said to have a more favorable prognosis as compared to conventional PDAC.

Cytology
FNAB will produce a viscous material and, consequently, smears will have a background of thick mucin, many times covering the entire slide (Fig. 5b). Admixed glandular cells range from sheets of mildly atypical epithelial cells, seen in the aspirates from the lower-grade tumors, to single cells and small clusters of malignant-appearing glandular cells [35] (Fig. 5c). Malignant ductal cells may contain intracytoplasmic mucin [36] (Fig. 5d).

Key Cytological Features
- Thick background mucin
- Malignant glandular cells
- Few signet ring cells

Ancillary Studies
Colloid carcinomas express MUC1, MUC2, and CDX2, which are not significantly expressed in conventional PDAC.

Differential Diagnosis
Extracellular mucin can be seen in a variety of pancreatic/extrapancreatic lesions including IPMNs, mucinous cystic tumors (MCTs), cystic pancreatic endocrine tumors, pancreatic lymphoepithelial cysts, gastrointestinal duplication cysts, and metastatic adenocarcinomas with mucin production such as colon cancer. MCTs are more common in women, have a much better prognosis, and on radiographic studies communicate with the pancreatic ductal system. Cytologic findings in conjunction with radiographic findings, and the patient's past history of another neoplasm,

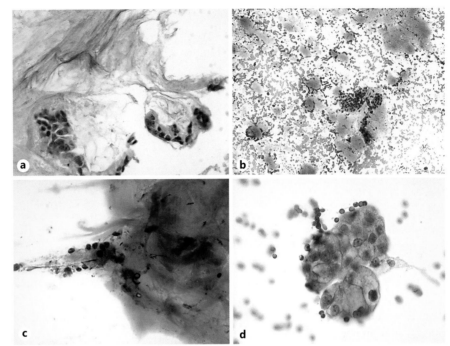

Fig. 5. Colloid carcinoma. **a** Strips of tumor cells floating in a background of mucin. HE stain, ×40. **b** Tumor admixed with an abundant background mucin. Diff-Quik stain, ×10. **c** Relatively bland-appearing cuboidal to low columnar tumor cells with mucin. Diff-Quik stain, ×40. **d** Exaggerated honeycomb appearance due to the presence of intracellular mucin. Papanicolaou stain, ×60.

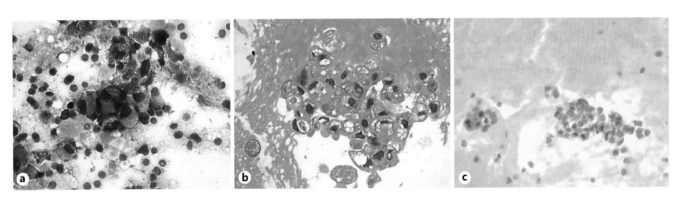

Fig. 6. SRCC. **a** Tumor cells with intracellular mucin vacuoles. Diff-Quik stain, ×60. **b** Cell block section with intracellular mucin pushing the tumor cell nuclei to the periphery. HE stain, ×60. **c** Special stain mucicarmine staining the intracellular mucin bright pink. Mucicarmine stain, ×40.

play an equally important role in making the correct diagnosis.

Signet Ring Cell Carcinoma
Histology
This is an extremely rare variant of PDAC (1%) in which survival and prognostic data are limited. Histologically, the tumor is composed of neoplastic cells with abundant intracytoplasmic mucin, either forming small aggregates or infiltrating singly. The cytomorphology is indistinguishable from that of SRCC from other sites. The tumor cells are most commonly found singly and when they comprise ≥50% of the tumor, the tumor is classified as an SRCC. This variant can be found in association with PDAC, conventional type [37].

Cytology
FNA smears show tumor cells with prominent cytoplasmic mucin vacuoles filling the cytoplasm and indenting the nuclei. A variable amount of mucin is present in the background (Fig. 6a, b).

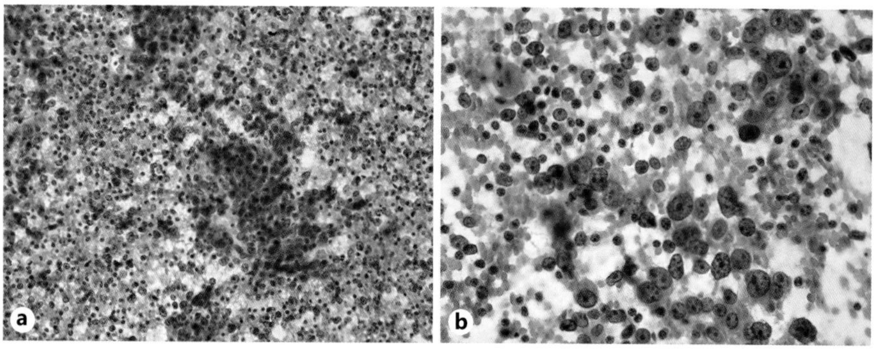

Fig. 7. Medullary carcinoma. **a** Loose groups and scattered tumor cells admixed with dense chronic inflammatory cell infiltrate. HE stain, ×20. **b** Tumor cells with round nuclei and prominent nucleoli admixed with numerous lymphocytes. HE stain, ×40.

Key Cytological Features
- Signet ring cells floating in pools of mucin
- Signet ring cells may be present singly or in loose clusters
- Component of conventional PDAC may be present

Ancillary Studies
Special stain mucicarmine highlights the intracellular mucin present (Fig. 6c). One of the studies [37] showed SRCC cells to be positive for cytokeratin AE1/3, cytokeratin CAM5.2, CK7, CK8, CK18, CK19, CEA, epithelial membrane antigen, p53, MUC1, and MUC5AC, and negative for CK20 and CDX2.

Differential Diagnosis
Signet ring cells can be confused with macrophages and inflammatory cells. However, demonstration of intracellular mucin by special stains such as mucicarmine and identifying the signet ring cells as epithelial (positive for cytokeratins) rather than inflammatory cells avoids this pitfall. A gastric or a breast primary should be excluded before diagnosing a primary pancreatic SRCC.

Medullary Carcinoma
Histology
Medullary carcinoma of the pancreas (MCP) is defined as a subtype of PDAC. MCP is histologically characterized by a syncytial growth pattern, poor gland formation, necrosis, and pushing tumor border with prominent intratumoral lymphocytes. Medullary carcinomas may arise sporadically or in patients with Lynch syndrome. This variant is said to have a better prognosis compared to conventional-type PDAC.

Cytology
Cytological features have not been specifically described for this variant, but cases are expected to recapitulate the histo-logic pattern of syncytial groups with eosinophilic cytoplasm being infiltrated by lymphocytes and plasma cells (Fig. 7a). Nuclear membranes have been observed to be smooth and nucleoli are prominent [38, 39] (Fig. 7b).

Key Cytological Features
- Malignant cells in syncytial groups
- Eosinophilic cytoplasm
- Lymphocytic infiltrate
- Necrotic background can be present

Ancillary Studies
The infiltrating lymphocytes react positive for immunostain CD3. There are two possible genetic pathways that have been described in the development of MCP. Mutations in *KRAS* and *BRAF* have been described in MCP. All the tumors exhibiting *KRAS* mutation are reported to be microsatellite stable. MSI has been reported in a few cases of MCP [39, 40].

Differential Diagnosis
Since cytologic features are not well established for this variant, many cases may be diagnosed as conventional-type PDAC. MCP may resemble acinar cell carcinoma (ACC). However, unlike ACC, the tumor cells in MCP will stain negative for trypsin and chymotrypsin.

Hepatoid Carcinoma
Histology
Hepatoid carcinoma appears histologically similar to hepatocellular carcinoma. This is a rare but aggressive variant of pancreatic adenocarcinoma. Hepatoid carcinomas may arise in a variety of extrahepatic sites, such as the pancreas, stomach, lung, gallbladder, ovary, and colon [41–43]. Clinically, the patients are middle aged or older and may present with elevated serum alpha-fetoprotein levels. The tumor

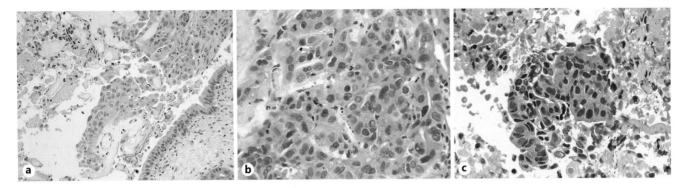

Fig. 8. Oncocytic carcinoma. **a** Intraductal portion of oncocytic carcinoma. HE stain, ×20. **b** Tumor cells with numerous intranuclear pseudoin-clusions. HE stain, ×40. **c** Cell block section showing tumor cells with an abundant eosinophilic and granular cytoplasm. HE stain, ×60.

may arise either as a solitary neoplasm or in combination with other pancreatic tumors such as neuroendocrine tumors, acinar, ductal, and mucinous adenocarcinomas. Histological examination reveals polygonal tumor cells with abundant eosinophilic granular cytoplasm with a trabecular and acinar growth pattern, in which bile formation may be present [44].

Cytology

Cytology smears are cellular with epithelioid tumor cells with round nuclei and an abundant cytoplasm [45]. Some of the tumor cells may contain bile.

Key Cytological Features

- Cellular smears with epithelioid cells that may contain bile
- Round nuclei with abundant, granular cytoplasm

Ancillary Studies

Hepatoid carcinomas stain positive for immunostains such as alpha-fetoprotein and hepatocyte antigen just like hepatocellular carcinomas. These tumors stain negative for neuroendocrine markers synaptophysin and chromogranin.

Differential Diagnosis

Metastatic hepatocellular carcinoma (HCC) is a close differential diagnosis that needs to be excluded. It is rare for HCC to metastasize to the pancreas but when it does it is usually at an advanced stage. Clinical history and imaging are critical to exclude a metastasis as the morphology and immunoprofile may overlap between the two. Other primary pancreatic neoplasms, such as neuroendocrine tumors, acinar cell carcinoma, intraductal oncocytic papillary neo-

plasm, and poorly differentiated PDAC, should be considered in the differential diagnosis. These entities can be distinguished by their characteristic morphology and immunoprofile, as discussed in other chapters.

Oncocytic Carcinoma

Oncocytic carcinoma of the pancreas is a rare variant of PDAC that arises from the oncocytic subtype of IPMN (IPMN-O) [46]. It is not considered a separate subtype of pancreatic ductal carcinoma according to WHO 2019 (5th edition) as its clinical and biological significance is not currently well defined. Patients with oncocytic carcinoma are said to have significantly better outcomes compared to those with classical PDAC [47, 48].

Histology

On histological examination, the tumor forms a large cystic mass. The cysts contain solid to papillary excrescences. The cysts are lined by simple columnar cells with abundant eosinophilic, granular cytoplasm (Fig. 8a). The nuclei are rounded with prominent nucleoli, intranuclear inclusions, and nuclear grooves (Fig. 8b).

Cytology

Cytological smears are characterized by tumor cells arranged in groups and papillae. Individual tumor cells are cuboidal to columnar and have abundant granular and eosinophilic cytoplasm (Fig. 8c). The nuclei are round with prominent nucleoli. The nuclear chromatin is pale. Nuclei have grooves and pseudoinclusions [49]. Necrosis has been occasionally reported.

Key Cytological Features

- Oncocytic tumor cells with abundant granular, eosinophilic cytoplasm
- Round nuclei with prominent nucleoli
- Nuclear grooves and pseudoinclusions

Ancillary Studies

The tumor cells stain positive for MUC1 and MUC6 and stain negative for neuroendocrine markers like synaptophysin and chromogranin. Oncocytic subtypes have a distinct pathway of tumorigenesis that likely contributes to the relatively indolent nature of the lesion. Unlike PDAC and the majority of IPMNs, this tumor is reported to be negative for *KRAS*, *CDKN2A*, *TP53*, *MADH4*, and *GNAS* mutations. Instead, molecular studies have shown somatic mutations in *ARHGAP26*, *ASXL1*, *EPHA8*, and *ERBB4* [50].

Differential Diagnosis

These tumors have to be differentiated from the oncocytic variant of neuroendocrine tumors. Nuclear features are very helpful in making this distinction besides immunostains. Nuclear grooves and pseudoinclusions are seen in oncocytic carcinomas and not in oncocytic variants of neuroendocrine tumors. Single cells, plasmacytoid cells, and naked cells are more commonly seen in neuroendocrine tumors. Immunostains for neuroendocrine differentiation such as synaptophysin and chromogranin are negative in oncocytic carcinoma. ACC, also in the differential, will usually stain for trypsin and chymotrypsin that helps in distinguishing it from oncocytic carcinoma.

Disclosure Statement

The authors have no conflicts of interest to disclose.

References

1 Porta M, Fabregat X, Malats N, Guarner L, Carrato A, de Miguel A, Ruiz L, Jariod M, Costafreda S, Coll S, Alguacil J, Corominas JM, Solà R, Salas A, Real FX. Exocrine pancreatic cancer: symptoms at presentation and their relation to tumour site and stage. Clin Transl Oncol 2005;7:189–197.

2 Chari ST; Leibson CL; Rabe KG; Ransom J; de Andrade M; Petersen GM: Probability of pancreatic cancer following diabetes: a population-based study. Gastroenterology 2005;129:504–511.

3 Stapley S, Peters TJ, Neal RD, Rose PW, Walter FM, Hamilton W: The risk of pancreatic cancer in symptomatic patients in primary care: a large case-control study using electronic records. Br J Cancer 2012;106:1940–1944.

4 Rückert F, Pilarsky C, Grützmann R: Serum tumor markers in pancreatic cancer – recent discoveries. Cancers 2010;2:1107–1124.

5 Tian F, Appert HE, Myles J, Howard JM: Prognostic value of serum CA 19–9 levels in pancreatic adenocarcinoma. Ann Surg 1992;215:350–355.

6 Tempero MA, Uchida E, Takasaki H, Burnett DA, Steplewski Z, Pour PM: Relationship of carbohydrate antigen 19–9 and Lewis in pancreatic cancer. Cancer Res 1987;47:5501–5503.

7 Duffy MJ, Sturgeon C, Lamerz R, Haglund C, Holubec VL, Klapdor R, Nicolini A, Topolcan O, Heinemann V: Tumor markers in pancreatic cancer: a European Group on Tumor Markers (EGTM) status report. Ann Oncol 2010;21:441–447.

8 Robins DB, Katz RL, Evans DB, Atkinson EN, Green L: Fine needle aspiration of the pancreas. In quest of accuracy. Acta Cytol 1995;39:1–10.

9 Lin F, Staerkel G: Cytologic criteria for well differentiated adenocarcinoma of the pancreas in fine-needle aspiration biopsy specimens. Cancer 2003;99:44–50.

10 Cohen MB, Egerter DP, Holly EA, Ahn DK, Miller TR: Pancreatic adenocarcinoma: regression analysis to identify improved cytologic criteria. Diagn Cytopathol 1991;7:341–345.

11 Chi Z, Wu HH, Cramer H, Lin J, Chen S: Cytomorphological features useful to prevent errors in the diagnosis of pancreatic adenocarcinoma by fine needle aspiration cytology. Acta Cytol 2017;61:7–16.

12 Eltoum IA, Eloubeidi MA, Chhieng DC, Tamhane A, Crowe R, Jhala D, St John KD, Wilcox CM, Siegal GP, Vickers S, Jhala NC: Cytologic grade independently predicts survival of patients with pancreatic adenocarcinoma. Am J Clin Pathol 2005;124:697–707.

13 Garcea G, Neal CP, Pattenden CJ, Steward WP, Berry DP: Molecular prognostic markers in pancreatic cancer: a systematic review. Eur J Cancer 2005;41:2213–2236.

14 Wang Y, Gao J, Li Z, Jin Z, Gong Y, Man X: Diagnostic value of mucins (MUC1, MUC2 and MUC5AC) expression profile in endoscopic ultrasound-guided fine-needle aspiration specimens of the pancreas. Int J Cancer 2007;121:2716–2722.

15 Ali S, Cohen C, Little JV, Sequeira JH, Mosunjac MB, Siddiqui MT: The utility of SMAD4 as a diagnostic immunohistochemical marker for pancreatic adenocarcinoma, and its expression in other solid tumors. Diagn Cytopathol 2007;35:644–648.

16 Hahn SA, Schutte M, Hoque AT, Moskaluk CA, da Costa LT, Rozenblum E, Weinstein CL, Fischer A, Yeo CJ, Hruban RH, Kern SE: DPC4, a candidate tumor suppressor gene at human chromosome 18q21.1. Science 1996;271:350–353.

17 Wachter DL, Schlabrakowski A, Hoegel J, Kristiansen G, Hartmann A, Riener MO: Diagnostic value of immunohistochemical IMP3 expression in core needle biopsies of pancreatic ductal adenocarcinoma. Am J Surg Pathol 2011;35:873–877.

18 Centeno BA: Pancreatic cytopathology: practical points to avoid common pitfalls. Evolving concepts in pancreatic pathology. USCAP Annual Meeting, San Antonio, 2011.

19 Jarboe EA, Layfield LJ: Cytologic features of pancreatic intraepithelial neoplasia and pancreatitis: potential pitfalls in the diagnosis of pancreatic ductal carcinoma. Diagn Cytopathol 2011;39:575–581.

20 Stelow EB, Pambuccian SE, Bardales RH, Debol SM, Mallery S, Lai R, Stanley MW: The cytology of pancreatic foamy gland adenocarcinoma. Am J Clin Pathol 2004;121:893–897.

21 Dursun N, Feng J, Basturk O, Bandyopadhyay S, Cheng JD, Adsay VN: Vacuolated cell pattern of pancreatobiliary adenocarcinoma: a clinicopathological analysis of 24 cases of a poorly recognized distinctive morphologic variant important in the differential diagnosis. Virchows Arch 2010;457:643–649.

22 Samad A, Conway AB, Attam R, Jessurun J, Pambuccian SE: Cytologic features of pancreatic adenocarcinoma with "vacuolated cell pattern." Report of a case diagnosed by endoscopic ultrasound-guided fine-needle aspiration. Diagn Cytopathol 2014;42:302–307.

23 Adsay V, Logani S, Sarkar F, Crissman J, Vaitkevicius V: Foamy gland pattern of pancreatic ductal adenocarcinoma: a deceptively benign-appearing variant. Am J Surg Pathol 2000;24:493–504.

24 Madura JA, Jarman BT, Doherty MG, Yum MN, Howard TJ: Adenosquamous carcinoma of the pancreas. Arch Surg 1999;134:599–603.

25 Trikudanathan G, Dasanu CA: Adenosquamous carcinoma of the pancreas: a distinct clinicopathologic entity. South Med J 2010;103:903–910.

26 Rahemtullah A, Misdraji J, Pitman MB: Adenosquamous carcinoma of the pancreas: cytologic features in 14 cases. Cancer 2003;99:372–378.

27 Brody JR, Costantino CL, Potoczek M, Cozzitorto J, McCue P, Yeo CJ, Hruban RH, Witkiewicz AK: Adenosquamous carcinoma of the pancreas harbors KRAS2, DPC4 and TP53 molecular alterations similar to pancreatic ductal adenocarcinoma. Mod Pathol 2009;22:651–659.

28 Paal E, Thompson LD, Frommelt RA, Przygodzki RM, Heffess CS: A clinicopathologic and immunohistochemical study of 35 anaplastic carcinomas of the pancreas with a review of the literature. Ann Diagn Pathol 2001;5:129–140.

29 Yorulmaz E, Kizilgül M, Özçelık S: Anaplastic pancreas carcinoma diagnosed by fine needle aspiration biopsy technique. Turk J Gastroenterol 2011;22:361–362.

30 Silverman JF, Dabbs DJ, Finley JL, Geisinger KR: Fine-needle aspiration biopsy of pleomorphic (giant cell) carcinoma of the pancreas. Cytologic, immunocytochemical, and ultrastructural findings. Am J Clin Pathol 1988;89:714–720.

31 Abbas S, Florian H, Judith F, Inga-Marie S, Philipp S, Arndt H, Robert S, Gunter K: Pancreatic undifferentiated rhabdoid carcinoma: KRAS alterations and SMARCB1 expression status define two subtypes. Mod Pathol 2015;28:248–260.

32 Layfield LJ, Bentz J: Giant-cell containing neoplasms of the pancreas: an aspiration cytology study. Diagn Cytopathol 2008;36:238–244.

33 Gao L, Li ZS, Jin ZD, Man XH, Zhang MH, Zhu MH: Undifferentiated carcinoma with osteoclast-like giant cells of the pancreas diagnosed by endoscopic ultrasonography-guided fine-needle aspiration. Chin Med J 2009;122:1598–1600.

34 Waters JA, Schnelldorfer T, Aguilar-Saavedra JR, Chen JH, Yiannoutsos CT, Lillemoe KD, Farnell MB, Sarr MG, Schmidt CM: Survival after resection for invasive intraductal papillary mucinous neoplasm and for pancreatic adenocarcinoma: a multi-institutional comparison according to American Joint Committee on Cancer Stage. J Am Coll Surg 2011;213:275–283.

35 Stelow EB, Shami VM, Abbott TE, Kahaleh M, Adams RB, Bauer TW, Debol SM, Abraham JM, Mallery S, Policarpio-Nicolas ML: The use of fine needle aspiration cytology for the distinction of pancreatic mucinous neoplasia. Am J Clin Pathol 2008;129:67–74.

36 Adsay NV, Pierson C, Sarkar F, Abrams J, Weaver D, Conlon KC, Brennan MF, Klimstra DS: Colloid (mucinous noncystic) carcinoma of the pancreas. Am J Surg Pathol 2001;25:26–42.

37 Terada T: Primary signet-ring cell carcinoma of the pancreas diagnosed by endoscopic retrograde pancreatic duct biopsy: a case report with an immunohistochemical study. Endoscopy 2012; 44(suppl 2):E141–E142.

38 Mitchell ML, Carney CN: Cytologic criteria for the diagnosis of pancreatic carcinoma. Am J Clin Pathol 1985;83:171–176.

39 Banville N, Geraghty R, Fox E, Leahy DT, Green A, Keegan D, Geoghegan J, O'Donoghue D, Hyland J, Sheahan K: Medullary carcinoma of the pancreas in a man with hereditary nonpolyposis colorectal cancer due to a mutation of the MSH2 mismatch repair gene. Hum Pathol 2006;37:1498–1502.

40 Yago A, Furuya M, Mori R, et al: Medullary carcinoma of the pancreas radiologically followed up as a cystic lesion for 9 years: a case report and review of the literature. Surg Case Rep 2018;4:80.

41 Steen S, Wolin E, Geller SA, Colquhoun S: Primary hepatocellular carcinoma ("hepatoid" carcinoma) of the pancreas: a case report and review of the literature. Clin Case Rep 2013;1:66–71.

42 Søreide JA, Greve OJ, Gudlaugsson E, Størset S: Hepatoid adenocarcinoma of the stomach – proper identification and treatment remain a challenge. Scand J Gastroenterol 2016;51:646–653.

43 Su JS, Chen YT, Wang RC, Wu CY, Lee SW, Lee TY: Clinicopathological characteristics in the differential diagnosis of hepatoid adenocarcinoma: a literature review. World J Gastroenterol 2013;19: 321–327.

44 Kuo PC, Chen SC, Shyr YM, et al: Hepatoid carcinoma of the pancreas. World J Surg Oncol 2015; 13:185.

45 Changa JM, Katariyaa NN, Lam-Himlinb DM, Haakinsona DJ, Ramanathanc RK, Halfdanarsonc TR, Boradc MJ, Pannalad R, Faigeld D, Mossa AA, Mathura AK: Hepatoid carcinoma of the pancreas: case report, next-generation tumor profiling, and literature review. Case Rep Gastroenterol 2016;10: 605–612.

46 Mino-Kenudson M, Fernández-del Castillo C, Baba Y, Valsangkar NP, Liss AS, Hsu M, Correa-Gallego C, Ingkakul T, Perez Johnston R, Turner BG, Androutsopoulos V, Deshpande V, McGrath D, Sahani DV, Brugge WR, Ogino S, Pitman MB, Warshaw AL, Thayer SP: Prognosis of invasive intraductal papillary mucinous neoplasm depends on histological and precursor epithelial subtypes. Gut 2011;60:1712–1720.

47 Chiang KC, Yu CC, Chen JR, Huang YT, Huang CC, Yeh CN, Tsai CS, Chen LW, Chen HC, Hsu JT, Wang CH, Chen HY: Oncocytic-type intraductal papillary mucinous neoplasm (IPMN)-derived invasive oncocytic pancreatic carcinoma with brain metastasis – a case report. World J Surg Oncol 2012;10:138.

48 Nozawa Y, Abe M, Sakuma H, Ogata M, Haga J, Sakuma H, Wakasa H: A case of pancreatic oncocytic tumor. Acta Pathol Jpn 1990;40:367–370.

49 Zhao Y, Bui MM, Allam-Nandyala P, Centeno BA: Fine-needle aspiration biopsy diagnosis of oncocytic carcinoma of the pancreas: a case report and literature review. Pathol Case Rev 2015;20:196–201.

50 Shows J, Bartsch C, Carmichael H, Qureshi I, Edil B, Fenton H: Molecular, histologic, and radiologic findings of high-grade invasive adenocarcinoma arising in oncocytic subtype of intraductal papillary mucinous neoplasm: a case report and review of literature. J Pancreat Cancer 2017;3.1:5–9.

Dr. Jasreman Dhillon
Moffitt Cancer Center
12902 USF Magnolia Drive
Tampa, FL 33612 (USA)
jasreman.dhillon@moffitt.org

Published online: September 29, 2020

Centeno BA, Dhillon J (eds): Pancreatic Tumors. Monogr Clin Cytol. Basel, Karger, 2020, vol 26, pp 92–108 (DOI:10.1159/000455737)

Non-Ductal Tumors of the Pancreas

Jasreman Dhillon

Department of Anatomic Pathology, Moffitt Cancer Center, Tampa, FL, USA; Department of Oncologic Sciences and Pathology, University of South Florida, Tampa, FL, USA

Abstract

Non-ductal tumors of the pancreas are relatively rare tumors and include pancreatic neuroendocrine tumors (PanNETs), poorly differentiated neuroendocrine carcinomas, acinar cell carcinoma, solid pseudopapillary neoplasm, and pancreatoblastoma. These tumors have a morphology and biology that is distinct from that of ductal neoplasms of the pancreas. PanNETs are the most common tumors among this group. A brief summary of each tumor is described here with an emphasis on the clinical presentation, cytological features, tumor histology, and immunohistochemical profile. Differential diagnoses for each entity are also discussed.   © 2020 S. Karger AG, Basel

Pancreatic Neuroendocrine Tumor

Pancreatic neuroendocrine tumors (PanNETs) are described in the WHO 2010 classification of gastrointestinal neuroendocrine tumors as neoplasms arising in the pancreas that predominantly have neuroendocrine differentiation [1]. PanNETs include well-differentiated neuroendocrine tumors and poorly differentiated neuroendocrine carcinomas (PDNECs), which will be described separately. PanNETs are relatively rare tumors that account for 2% of all the

pancreatic neoplasms [2]. These tumors are derived and composed of epithelial cells that show neuroendocrine differentiation. Most of these tumors are speculated to arise from neuroendocrine-type cells that reside in the pancreatic ductal epithelium and not from the islets of Langerhans [3]. The nomenclature, grading, and staging of PanNETs were standardized and updated within the last decade. The term 'neuroendocrine tumor' was adopted by the WHO 2010 classification system which classified them according to differentiation and grade [1]. PanNETs were classified as well-differentiated or poorly differentiated, the latter morphologically being NECs. The grade was based on mitotic activity and the Ki-67 labeling index. A problem with this original version of the classification is that it lumped well-differentiated PanNET grade 3 with PDNECs as high grade based on the proliferative index. The grading system has been recently updated to reflect the difference in biology between grade 3 PanNETs and PDNECs. PanNETs are well-differentiated neuroendocrine tumors that maintain their cytoplasmic differentiation. According to the WHO 2017 classification, PanNETs are divided into grade 1, grade 2, and grade 3. PDNECs are no longer graded. Grade 1 PanNETs are well-differentiated tumors with a mitotic count of <2/10 high-power fields (HPF) and Ki-67 <3%. Grade 2 PanNETs are well-differentiated tumors with a mitotic count of 2–20/10 HPF

Table 1. WHO 2017 classification system for PanNETs

WHO nomenclature	Grade	Traditional nomenclature	Mitoses/10 HPF	Ki-67 proliferation index, %
Well-differentiated PanNET	1	Carcinoid, islet cell tumor	<2	<3
Well-differentiated PanNET	2	Atypical carcinoid, islet cell tumor	2–20	3–20
Well-differentiated PanNET	3	Poorly differentiated neuroendocrine carcinoma	>20	>20

and Ki-67 3–20%. There is a small group of well-differentiated PanNETs with a Ki-67 index >20% and a mitotic rate >20/10 HPF. In WHO 2010, these tumors were considered as grade 3 PDNECs. However, they have a typical morphology of well-differentiated neuroendocrine tumors and are not as aggressive as PDNECs but are more aggressive than grade 2 PanNETs [4]. In addition, these tumors do not have the genetic abnormalities seen in PDNECs and, unlike PDNECs, they are less responsive to platinum-based chemotherapy [5, 6]. In the WHO 2017 blue book of endocrine tumors and AJCC 8th edition, these tumors are classified as grade 3 well-differentiated neuroendocrine tumors [7].

The WHO 2017 classification system for PanNETs and their comparison with the traditional nomenclature is provided in Table 1. Grading according to the mitotic and Ki-67 indices can sometimes be discordant. In such instances, the recommendation is to assign the higher grade [8]. The Ki-67 needs to be assessed in at least 500 cells, in areas designated as hot spots. Mitoses should be counted in 50 HPF and reported per 10 HPF, which should equal a 2-mm^2 area. A quantitative assessment, and not eyeballing, is recommended [9].

The WHO recommendations for grading of PanNETs have not been established for cytological specimens. FNA cytology samples carry several limitations, predominantly due to sample size and selective sampling in a heterogenous tumor. There can be both understaging and upstaging of PanNETs in cytology, especially understaging [7]. However, different studies have shown that WHO grading of PanNETs, when performed on cytologic samples by assessing the Ki-67 index on cell block material, shows good correlation with the surgical resection specimens [10, 11].

Clinical Presentation
PanNETs commonly occur in adults between the age of 30 and 60 years. Men and women are equally affected [3]. PanNETs are rarely seen in children and adolescents, but when

present are usually associated with a genetic/familial [12] predisposition such as multiple endocrine neoplasia 1 (MEN1), tuberous sclerosis, von Hippel-Lindau (VHL) disease, and neurofibromatosis. Non-functioning PanNETs occur more commonly in the head of the pancreas [13, 14]. However, PanNETs can occur anywhere in the pancreas. PanNETs may be identified because of symptoms related to the increased secretion of endocrine hormones such as insulin, gastrin, glucagon, vasoactive intestinal peptide (VIP), and somatostatin from tumor cells. Insulinomas are the most common cause of functional syndromes, followed by gastrinomas, glucagonomas, VIPomas, somatostatinomas, in PanNETs [15, 16]. Insulinomas are small tumors that secrete insulin and present with autonomic symptoms such as palpitations, tremor, sweating, hunger, and neuroglycopenic symptoms, such as weakness, confusion, agitation, blurred vision, seizures, or hypoglycemic coma [17]. Gastrinomas secrete gastrin and are associated with Zollinger-Ellison syndrome, which is characterized by increased acid production by the stomach leading to severe and extensive peptic ulcer disease. Gastrinomas are the most common functioning PanNETs in patients with MEN1 syndrome. Most pancreatic glucagonomas are malignant and present with necrolytic migratory erythema, diabetes mellitus, anemia, weight loss, diarrhea, venous thrombosis, and neuropsychiatric symptoms such as ataxia, dementia, optic atrophy, and proximal muscle weakness. VIPomas produce VIP and the majority of tumors have metastasized by the time of diagnosis. Excessive amounts of VIP produce a large volume of watery diarrhea with dehydration, hypokalemia, achlorhydria, and metabolic acidosis [18]. The majority of somatostatin-secreting tumors are malignant and are usually diagnosed by immunohistochemical staining of the granules. Rare functional PanNETs may secrete pancreatic polypeptide, calcitonin, adrenocorticotropic hormone, parathyroid hormone-related protein, serotonin, luteinizing hormone, renin, and erythropoietin.

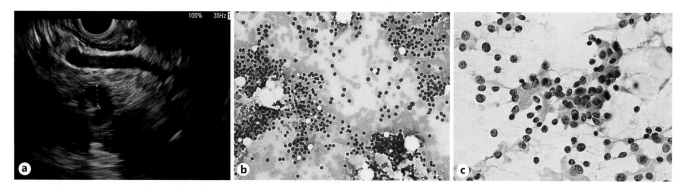

Fig. 1. PanNET. **a** EUS image of a 3.5-cm PanNET present in the head of the pancreas abutting the superior mesenteric vein. **b** PanNET with monomorphic tumor cells present as diffuse sheets and forming rosettes (upper right-hand corner). Diff-Quik stain, ×20. **c** PanNET cells exhibiting a salt and pepper chromatin pattern. Papanicolaou stain, ×60.

However, the majority of PanNETs are non-functioning tumors [18] and may not secrete any hormones, making them difficult to detect and leading to their identification in late stages of disease secondary to obstruction or abdominal discomfort such as abdominal pain, anorexia, weight loss, and nausea related to the growing mass [19]. Non-functioning PanNETs secrete a number of substances such as chromogranins, neuron-specific enolase, and pancreatic polypeptide that do not present clinically with a hormonal syndrome. Many non-functioning tumors are detected as incidental findings on radiology.

Endocrine testing, imaging, and histological evidence are all required to accurately diagnose PanNETs. Elevated serum levels of corresponding hormones are usually present in functioning PanNETs. If hormonal hypersecretion syndrome is suspected, appropriate biochemical testing is performed to determine hormonal hypersecretion and followed by imaging, endoscopy, and biopsy. Chromogranin A, neuron-specific enolase, and pancreastatin are the most useful PanNET markers in serum [20–22]. Fasting levels of pancreatic polypeptide, gastrin, proinsulin, insulin, glucagon, and VIP are frequently elevated in functioning PanNETs. Blood collected from hypoglycemic episodes of patients with insulinoma shows inappropriately high insulin and C-peptide serum levels.

Imaging Studies
Computed tomography (CT) or magnetic resonance imaging (MRI) of the abdomen and pelvis is important to evaluate the extent of disease in the pancreas and to evaluate for liver, lymph node, and peritoneal metastases. Imaging studies, as described in the chapter by Morse and Klapman [this

vol., pp. 21–33], typically show a hypervascular well-circumscribed pancreatic mass (Fig. 1a). Somatostatin receptor functional imaging is one of the main techniques used for the evaluation of neuroendocrine tumors [23]. The most used is indium In-111 (^{111}In)-pentetreotide SPECT (single-photon emission CT), most commonly known by the trade name OctreaScan. Recently, ^{111}In-pentetreotide has been largely superseded by the ^{68}Ga-labeled somatostatin receptor analogs DOTATATE, DOTATOC, and DOTANOC.

Histology
Sporadic cases of PanNET present as well-circumscribed, solitary masses which can involve any part of the pancreas, but occur more commonly in the head of the pancreas. On gross examination, these tumors are soft and fleshy due to abundant cellularity and without a stromal reaction. Although most of the PanNETs are solid, about 5% may be cystic [3]. On microscopic examination, PanNETs form sheets of stroma-poor tumor cells, this feature being typical of all non-ductal neoplasms of the pancreas. The tumor cells form cords, nests, trabeculae, and pseudorosettes, and are monomorphic with round to oval nuclei with salt and pepper chromatin. The cytoplasm may vary in amount. It may be scant, or it may be eccentric imparting a plasmacytoid appearance. There is usually no necrosis. When present, necrosis is focal and involves single cells or may be comedo-like. The mitotic activity and proliferation rate, as determined by the Ki-67 labeling index, predicts the grade of the tumor.

Morphologic variants of PanNETs include the lipid-rich or clear cell variant [24] which may resemble renal cell carcinoma or an adrenocortical tumor, the oncocytic variant

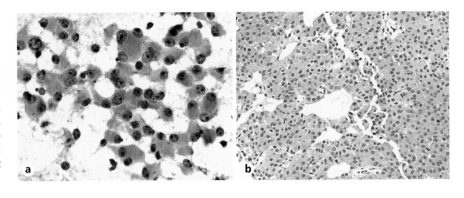

Fig. 2. Oncocytic variant of PanNET. **a** The cells have an abundant, well-defined oncocytic cytoplasm. The nuclei are round and uniform, with prominent nucleoli, some cells are binucleated. Papanicolaou stain, ×60. **b** The cell block shows cells with an abundant granular cytoplasm with distinct cell borders, and round nuclei with prominent nucleoli. HE stain, ×20.

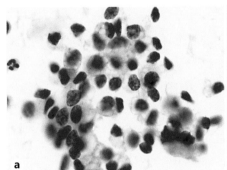
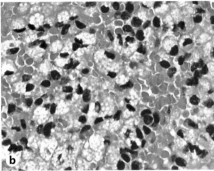
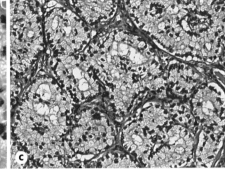

Fig. 3. Clear cell variant of PanNET. **a** Cluster of tumor cells with round to oval nuclei and a granular chromatin pattern and moderate amount of cytoplasm containing numerous small sharply demarcated vacuoles. Papanicolaou stain, ×60. **b** Cell block section with monomorphic tumor cells exhibiting a clear cytoplasm. HE stain, ×40. **c** Concurrent histology showing a well-differentiated PanNET with prominent clear cell change. HE stain, ×40. Images courtesy of Dr. Qiusheng Si (Mount Sinai Hospital, New York City, NY, USA).

[25], which resembles hepatocellular carcinoma, and the peliotic variant, which has abundant blood vessels and pools of blood. PanNETs with prominent rhabdoid [26] and signet ring cell features [27] and pigmented cells [28] have also been reported.

Cytology
FNA smears are often cellular. The smears show loosely cohesive clusters of epithelial cells in a background of a predominantly single cell population. Some of the clusters appear to form rosette-like structures (Fig. 1b). The tumor cells are small to medium, monomorphic, and often have a plasmacytoid appearance. The nuclei are round to oval with smooth nuclear membranes with granular, salt and pepper chromatin (Fig. 1c). Many bare nuclei may be present in the background as these cells are frequently stripped of their cytoplasm. The cytoplasm is amphophilic, and varies in density and quantity.

The variants of PanNET may be identified on FNA. The oncocytic variant of PanNET has tumor cells with abundant eosinophilic, granular cytoplasm, large round to oval nuclei with prominent nucleoli, and relatively smooth nuclear membranes (Fig. 2a, b) [25]. Clear cell PanNET is characterized by cells with abundant, multivacuolated cytoplasm (Fig. 3a–c) [29]. Clear cell PanNET can be sporadic or syndromic and is particularly associated with VHL syndrome [30, 31]. The rhabdoid variant has been described on FNA [32]. The cells have cytoplasmic inclusions that are pale on Papanicolaou and pink on Romanowsky stains. The inclusions may indent the nucleus, imparting a signet ring appearance (Fig. 4).

Key Cytological Features
- Cellular smears typically with a clean background
- Predominantly single and loosely cohesive clusters of monomorphic tumor cells
- Round to oval nuclei with smooth nuclear membrane contours

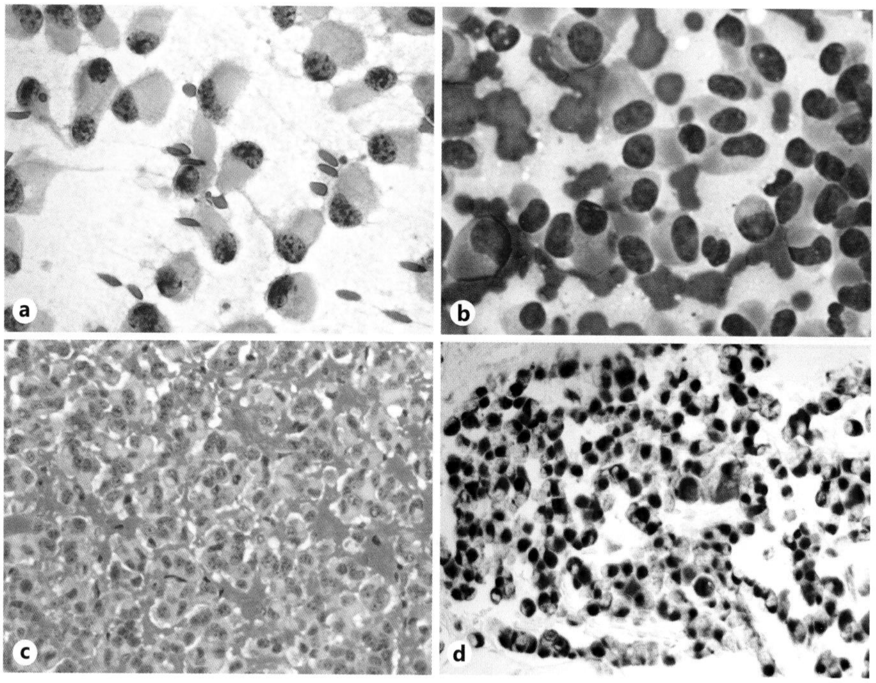

Fig. 4. PanNET with rhabdoid cells. **a** The cells have speckled chromatin and most contain a round, homogenously pale body within their cytoplasm. In some cells, the nucleus is indented by the pale body. Papanicolaou stain, ×60. **b** The intracytoplasmic bodies stain a pink color, distinct from the cytoplasm. Diff-Quik stain, ×60. **c** On histology, the inclusions are homogenously pink. HE stain, ×20. **d** AE/AE3 is intensely positive in the cytoplasmic globules. Immunoperoxidase stain, ×40. Images courtesy of Dr. Christopher VanDenBussche (Johns Hopkins Medical Institutions, Baltimore, MD, USA).

- Moderate to variable amount of eccentric cytoplasm in the typical PanNET
- Stripped nuclei
- Finely granular salt and pepper chromatin
- Variant morphologies will maintain the salt and pepper chromatin pattern and and rounded nuclear shape, but will have variable cytoplasmic features:
- clear cell – finely vacuolated, clear cytoplasm
- oncocytic – abundant, dense, eosinophilic cytoplasm, and prominent nucleoli
- pigmented – melanin pigment in cytoplasm
- rhabdoid – abundant densely eosinophilic cytoplasmic inclusions that displace the nuclei towards the periphery
- signet ring – single cytoplasmic vacuole

Ancillary Studies

PanNETs are positive for cytokeratins (CK) 8 and 18, AE1/AE3 and CAM 5.2, and neuroendocrine markers including neural cell adhesion marker (CD56), chromogranin A, and synaptophysin (Fig. 5a–d). The intracytoplasmic inclusions of the rhabdoid variant stain intensely with cytokeratins [32]. A novel immunohistochemical marker, insulinoma-associated protein 1 (INSM1), has been described for neuroendocrine neoplasms, which is a relatively sensitive and specific marker (Fig. 5e) [33]. Other markers that may be expressed by PanNET include PAX8, ISL1, PDX1, and CDX2 [34]. These may be useful for identification of PanNET at metastatic sites [34, 35].

Assessment of the mitotic count on FNA smears has not been validated and assessment on cell blocks is often not feasible due to the fragmented nature of the samples, which do not allow for counting of a continuous field. However, immunohistochemistry for Ki-67 can be readily performed on cell blocks and the cells expressing the Ki-67 counted to obtain a Ki-67 labeling index. A caveat is that the approach to evaluating Ki-67 has not been standardized, and the counts may be falsely low or high. A comment should be added to the cytology report stating that the grade may change on resection or follow-up histology.

Mutations in the genes *ATRX/DAXX* and *MEN1*, and in the mTOR pathway genes have been identified in PanNETs, but not in pancreatic NECs [36]. Immunohistochemistry will show loss of ATRX/DAXX protein in tumors harboring these mutations. Somatostatin receptor 2A (SSTR2A) has shown an inverse relationship with an increasing Ki-67 proliferation index, and is expressed in grade 1 and grade 2 tumors, but less expressed in grade 3 tumors and NECs [37]. Loss of expression of SSTR2 is therefore an indicator that the neoplasm is grade 3 PanNET or NEC.

Dhillon

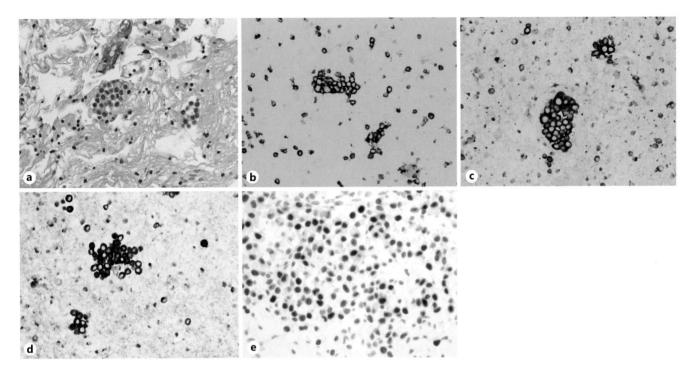

Fig. 5. Ancillary studies in PanNET. **a** Cell block section of PanNET showing loosely cohesive clusters and single cells of PanNET. HE stain, ×40. **b** The cells show strong cytoplasmic expression for pancytokeratin AE1/AE3. Immunoperoxidase stain, ×20. Synaptophysin (**c**) and chromogranin (**d**). Immunoperoxidase stain, ×20. **e** Nuclear expression for INSM1. Immunoperoxidase stain, ×40.

Differential Diagnosis

The most significant differential diagnosis is with other non-ductal neoplasms as described in the following sections. Other entities to consider include pancreatic ductal adenocarcinoma (PDAC), plasmacytoma, and metastases.

PanNET can be mistaken for PDAC when prominent nucleoli and nuclear pleomorphism are present, or if the cell sample is limited [38]. Often, the imaging findings may be suggestive of a PanNET. The nuclei of PanNET will retain their smooth nuclear outlines, compared to the nuclei of PDAC. Also, PDAC will show glandular differentiation, not seen in PanNETs. An example of a case of PanNET misinterpreted as adenocarcinoma is illustrated in Figure 6a–c.

Since PanNET has a plasmacytoid appearance, plasmacytoma enters the differential diagnosis. However, plasmacytoma in the pancreas would be very unusual. A plasmacytoid-appearing neoplasm in the pancreas should always be considered to be a PanNET until proven otherwise. Also, since PanNETs may have stripped nuclei, lymphoma enters the differential diagnosis. The presence of lymphoglandular bodies suggests the presence of lymphoma. PanNET may have elongated nuclei, similar to those seen in medullary carcinoma of the thyroid. In such cases, the elongated nuclei may bring up the differential diagnosis of a spindle cell neoplasm. However, the nuclei will retain their salt and pepper chromatin distribution.

Clear cell PanNET is characterized by cells with abundant, multivacuolated cytoplasm containing lipid [24]. This entity must be distinguished from other tumors involving the pancreas that can exhibit clear cell features such as PDAC, solid pseudopapillary neoplasm (SPN), acinar cell carcinoma (ACC), solid variant of serous cystadenoma, and metastatic tumors such as renal cell carcinoma. Usually, the main differential is with metastatic renal cell carcinoma. Metastatic renal cell carcinoma will show large nuclei with irregular nuclear membranes and prominent nucleoli. The nuclei of clear cell PanNET will retain the smooth nuclear membranes and salt and pepper chromatin.

Being aware of the existence of these variants and the utilization of an immunohistochemical panel will clarify the diagnosis. The tumor cells in PanNETs, both the usual and variant morphologies, are usually positive for pancytokeratins and the neuroendocrine markers INSM1, synaptophysin, and chromogranin A. When in doubt, it is best to utilize

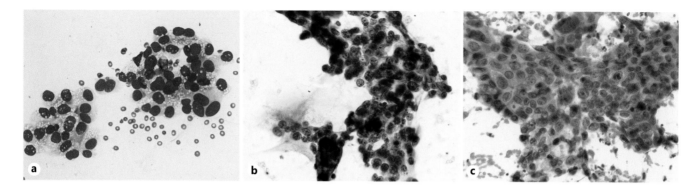

Fig. 6. A case of PanNET mistaken as adenocarcinoma. **a** Cluster of tumor cells with overlapping and round nuclei with smooth nuclear membranes and cytoplasmic vacuoles. Diff-Quik stain, ×40. **b** Mildly pleomorphic tumor cells with overlapping nuclei, prominent nucleoli, and a finely distributed chromatin pattern. Papanicolaou stain, ×40. **c** Cluster of mildly pleomorphic pancreatic adenocarcinoma cells with anisonucleosis and prominent nucleoli. Papanicolaou stain, ×60.

a panel, including neuroendocrine markers and differentiation specific to the differential diagnosis, to confirm the diagnosis.

Poorly Differentiated NECs

PDNECs of the pancreas are defined as neoplasms arising in the pancreas that have predominantly neuroendocrine differentiation and are divided into small- and large-cell NECs.

Clinical Presentation
PDNECs in the pancreas are rare, and typically occur in older patients. These tumors are extremely aggressive and have often disseminated at the time of diagnosis. They do not have any specific clinical features, and usually present with symptoms relating to a mass. PDNECs are more common in older men with a median survival of less than 2 years [3]. They are usually treated with platinum-based therapy and are no longer graded according to the 2017 WHO classification.

Histology
Based on the cell size, PDNEC are subdivided into small-cell and large-cell variants. The large-cell variant is more common and is composed of large cells with prominent nucleoli and variable cytoplasm. The small-cell variant shows small to intermediate cells with coarse salt and pepper chromatin, high nuclear-to-cytoplasmic ratio, inconspicuous nucleoli, prominent nuclear molding, and crush artifact. Mitotic activity is brisk (often >40/10 HPFs) and necrosis is often extensive in both of these subtypes. No reactivity for peptide hormones is found in PDNECs.

Cytology
The cytological features of a pancreatic small-cell NEC are similar to the lung counterpart. FNA samples are typically cellular with abundant background necrosis. Tumor cells are arranged singly, or in cohesive clusters or groups. They are small to intermediate in size (20 μm) and show extensive crush artifact. The nuclei are round, oval, spindled, or fusiform in shape. The cells have a high nuclear-to-cytoplasmic ratio, typically scant cytoplasm, and are cyanophilic on Papanicolaou stain (Fig. 7a–c). The chromatin is finely granular exhibiting a salt and pepper pattern. Mitotic activity is brisk. Large-cell NEC cells are larger in size (>30 μm) and have a variable amount of cytoplasm. The nuclei are rounded to oval, vesicular, and typically contain a central prominent nucleolus (Fig. 7d). Typically, the salt and pepper-like chromatin pattern is not present in these tumors and most often they are misdiagnosed as poorly differentiated adenocarcinoma.

Key Cytological Features
Small-Cell Carcinoma:
- Small cells up to 20 μm
- Scant cytoplasm
- Round, oval, spindled, or fusiform with nuclear molding, a high N/C ratio, and salt and pepper chromatin
- Associated with extensive crush artifact
- Abundant necrosis, including apoptotic cells
- Brisk mitotic activity

Large Cell NEC:
- Cells usually >30 μm
- Variable amount of cytoplasm

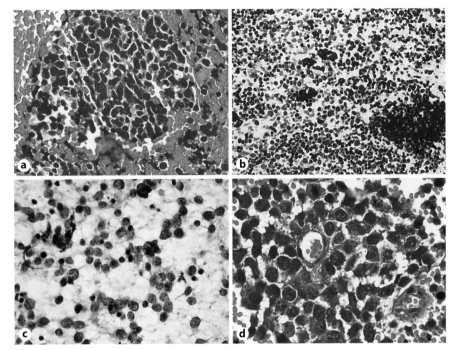

Fig. 7. PDNECs. **a** Small-cell carcinoma – cell block section showing molding of tumor cells. HE stain, ×40. **b** Small-cell carcinoma showing diffuse sheets of tumor cells with minimal cytoplasm and molding. Diff-Quik stain, ×20. **c** Small-cell carcinoma cells with a finely stippled chromatin pattern. Papanicolaou stain, ×60. **d** Large-cell NEC showing cells with prominent nucleoli and a moderate amount of cytoplasm. HE stain, ×40.

- Nuclei are vesicular with prominent nucleoli
- Abundant necrosis
- Brisk mitotic activity

Ancillary Studies

Cytokeratin is positive, usually in a dot-like pattern. No reactivity for peptide hormones is found in PDNECs. Large-cell NEC may stain positive for neuroendocrine markers. However, the staining is not as robust as in well-differentiated NETs. Small cell NECs may not express neuroendocrine markers at all. This does not preclude a diagnosis of small-cell NEC as long as other diagnostic entities are excluded. The Ki-67 proliferative index often exceeds 55% [6].

PDNECs harbor mutations on *TP53*, *KRAS*, *SMAD4*, and retinoblastoma gene (*RB1*). Immunohistochemical analysis for the corresponding proteins serves as a surrogate marker for mutations in these genes, with p53 showing a diffuse aberrant nuclear expression, and loss of SMAD4 and Rb protein. In cases in which Rb protein is retained, loss of p16 protein may be found [39]. As already described, SSTR2A shows an inverse relationship with an increasing Ki-67 labeling index. Most PDNECs lose expression for this protein. BCL2 protein is overexpressed in PDNECs, but not in PanNETs [5].

Differential Diagnosis

PDNECs have to be differentiated from well-differentiated grade 3 PanNETs. Cytologically, well-differentiated PanNETs usually have an abundant granular cytoplasm resulting in a low nuclear-to-cytoplasmic ratio and stippled chromatin. PDNECs have a less granular cytoplasm and a higher nuclear-to-cytoplasmic ratio, with either nuclei with open chromatin and conspicuous nucleoli (large-cell NEC) or hyperchromatic and molded nuclei lacking nucleoli (small cell carcinoma). In the presence of a coexisting conventional carcinoma (i.e., squamous cell carcinoma or adenocarcinoma) a high-grade neuroendocrine neoplasm should be considered a PDNEC. Immunohistochemical stains for p53, Rb1, ATRX/DAXX, and SSTR2A will be helpful for differentiating these as already described [39, 40].

Besides morphological features of PDNECs, as described above, neuroendocrine markers can be helpful in distinguishing them from PDACs. PDACs are negative for neuroendocrine markers. ACC cells exhibit a moderate amount of granular cytoplasm and a round nucleus with a prominent nucleolus that can be confused with large-cell NEC. However, large-cell NECs have relatively less granular cytoplasm and a higher nucleus-to-cytoplasmic ratio. Immunohistochemical stains can help distinguish the two entities as acinar cell carcinomas (ACCs) are positive for trypsin, chymotrypsin, and BCL10, whereas PDNECs are not.

Metastatic carcinomas from other organs should also be considered in the differential diagnosis. Clinical history, radiographic findings, and use of ancillary tests help to arrive at the correct diagnosis.

Mixed Neuroendocrine-Non-Neuroendocrine Neoplasms

The WHO 2019 defines these as neoplasms with multiple lines of differentiation based on morphology and immunohistochemistry. They consist of a neuroendocrine component with either an acinar or ductal component, or both. The secondary component must represent at least 30% of the neoplasm; therefore, an adequate cytological sample is required to make this diagnosis.

Acinar Cell Carcinoma

The WHO 2019 defines acinar cell carcinoma (ACC) as a malignant epithelial neoplasm composed of cells with morphological resemblance to acinar cells and with evidence of pancreatic exocrine enzyme production [41]. ACCs are rare and comprise <2% of the pancreatic tumors in adults and 15% of those in children [41]. Males are affected more frequently than females with a male-to-female ratio of 2.1:1.

The prognosis of ACC is intermediate between PanNETs and PDAC [42], with many patients presenting with liver metastases. ACCs are typically positive for trypsin and/or chymotrypsin, the exocrine enzymes produced by benign acinar cells.

Clinical Presentation
ACCs usually present with non-specific symptoms such as abdominal pain, weight loss, nausea and diarrhea. Jaundice can be present but is much rarer than in ductal adenocarcinomas. Up to 10–15% of patients may present with lipase hypersecretion syndrome [43], in which patients have an elevated blood level of lipase that is secreted by the tumor cells. Elevated levels of lipase in these patients cause subcutaneous fat necrosis and polyarthralgia.

Imaging
ACCs are generally large tumors that are relatively sharply circumscribed. These tumors enhance homogenously on CT scans. Cystic change secondary to necrosis can occur.

Histology
ACCs are more circumscribed than PDACs. They are very cellular tumors and lack the intervening desmoplastic stroma noted in PDACs and exhibit acinar, solid, less often trabecular, and/or gland-like architecture. The acinar pattern is the most common. The tumor cells are arranged in small acinar units with central lumina forming a cribriform or gland-like pattern. The second most common pattern is the solid pattern where the tumor cells are arranged in solid sheets separated by small vessels. The neoplastic cells have a moderate to abundant amount of eosinophilic to amphophilic cytoplasm that is finely granular. The nucleus is round to oval with a prominent nucleolus. The mitotic rate is variable but generally high.

Cytology
Smears from ACC are hypercellular with the presence of thick, 3-dimensional groups, clustered acini, trabeculae, and club-shaped arrangements of tumor cells (Fig. 8a–c) [44]. The tumor cells have an amphophilic to eosinophilic, granular cytoplasm, minimal pleomorphism, and nucleoli suggestive of acinar differentiation. The cytoplasmic granules in some cases may be sparse. Necrosis may be present. The cytological features of ACC mimic PanNET. ACC is often misdiagnosed as poorly differentiated adenocarcinoma of the pancreas [45].

Key Cytological Features
- Hypercellular smears with the presence of 3-dimensional groups and clustered acini
- The tumor cells are usually monomorphic
- Moderate to abundant granular cytoplasm
- Round to oval nucleus with a prominent nucleolus
- Zymogen granules in the cytoplasm, appear as negative images on Romanowsky stains

Ancillary Studies
The cytoplasmic zymogen granules in ACC are periodic acid-Schiff (PAS) positive and resistant to diastase digestion (dPAS). The tumor cells are positive for the immunohistochemical stains chymotrypsin and trypsin. ACCs are usually positive for CK8 and CK18 and less commonly show immunoreactivity for CK7, CK19, and CK20, traditionally known as markers of ductal adenocarcinomas [46]. BCL10 has been recently recognized to exhibit immunoreactivity in ACCs, where it is very helpful in diagnosing these tumors due to its high sensitivity and specificity [47]. Scattered neuroendocrine cells positive for chromogranin A or synapto-

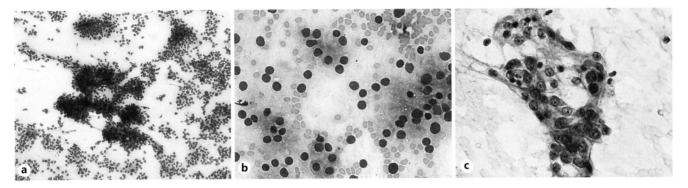

Fig. 8. ACC. **a** Hypercellular smear with cells present in loosely cohesive clusters and trabeculae. Diff-Quik stain, ×10. **b** Tumor cells forming acini with a moderate to abundant amount of amphophilic and granular cytoplasm. Diff-Quik, ×40. **c** Tumor cells with prominent nucleoli and a moderate amount of granular cytoplasm. Papanicolaou stain, ×60.

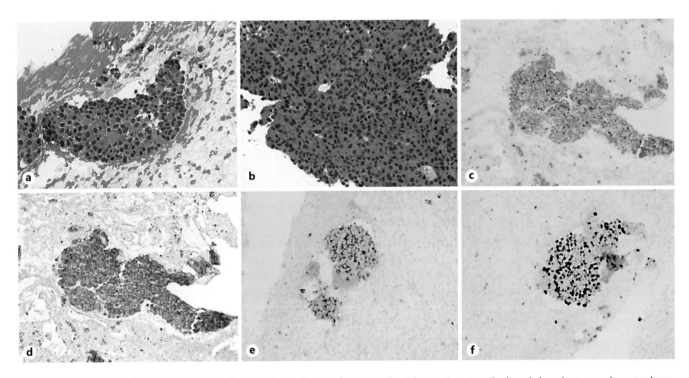

Fig. 9. ACC ancillary studies. **a** Cell block section showing a cluster of tumor cells with prominent nucleoli and abundant granular cytoplasm. HE stain, ×40. **b** PAS with diastase shows cytoplasmic granules, ×20. **c–f** Immunohistochemical stains on cell block sections. **c** Trypsin, ×20. **d** BCL10, ×20. **e** Chromogranin, ×20. **f** Ki-67, ×20.

physin, or both, may be present in ACCs (Fig. 9a–f). Nuclear expression of β-catenin can be found in about 10% of ACCs [41].

Differential Diagnosis
The differential diagnosis of ACC is broad and ranges from benign acinar cells, PanNET, solid pseudopapillary neo-

plasm (SPN), and PDAC to metastatic tumors. Overinterpretation of benign acinar cells as a neoplastic process should be avoided. The cellularity of normal pancreas with abundant normal acini may lead to the suspicion of ACC. Benign pancreatic acini typically form more prominent organoid arrangements of acini with retention of the normal acinar architecture. It may be difficult to distinguish ACC from Pan-

NET due to morphologic similarities and scattered positivity for neuroendocrine markers in ACC. Up to 40% of ACCs can have scattered neuroendocrine cells that can be positive for neuroendocrine markers [48, 49]. However, the presence of a high-mitotic index, abundant necrosis, and clearly evident nucleoli in apparently well to moderately differentiated cells with abundant eosinophilic cytoplasm, should give rise to the suspicion of an ACC that can be confirmed by the appropriate immunohistochemical stains as described above.

SPN is more frequent in females and rarely shows abundant necrosis. SPNs typically show nuclear immunoreactivity for β-catenin and strong expression of CD10 that can, however, also be found in about 10 and 60% of ACCs, respectively. For this reason, these two markers should not be used alone but in association with acinar-specific markers such as trypsin and BCL10 [50].

Mixed Acinar NECs

Acinar cell cancers with a substantial proportion (>30%) of more than one cell type are designated as mixed acinar carcinomas [41]. When the second component is neuroendocrine cells identified with immunohistochemical markers, it is classified as mixed acinar-NEC and follows an aggressive course similar to pure ACC [51]. This is different from mixed neuroendocrine-non-neuroendocrine neoplasms, in which the two cell types are recognized on morphology, not just immunohistochemical expression. When the ductal cells comprise a substantial second component, the tumors are classified as mixed acinar-ductal carcinoma. Mixed acinar-neuroendocrine-ductal carcinomas also occur, but are extremely rare. Recognition on cytology may be difficult and these mixed acinar tumors may be misclassified as Pan-NETs, pure ACCs, SPNs, and pancreatoblastoma.

Solid Pseudopapillary Neoplasm

The WHO 2019 defines SPN of the pancreas as a low-grade malignant neoplasm composed of poorly cohesive monomorphic epithelial cells forming solid and pseudopapillary structures. SPNs of the pancreas rare neoplasms that comprise approximately 1–2% of all pancreatic tumors [52].

Clinical Presentation
SPNs predominantly occur in women in the third and fourth decades of life [53]. These tumors are usually found incidentally on routine examination for another indication. Symptomatic tumors may present with abdominal discomfort, pain, nausea, and vomiting. Jaundice is rare. SPNs are typically localized to the pancreas although 10–15% may develop metastases to the liver and/or peritoneum [54]. Even with metastases, these tumors have a very good clinical outcome, with 5-year survival reported in up to 97% [55].

Imaging
Radiographic studies show a sharply demarcated, variably solid and cystic mass without internal septations involving the pancreas (Fig. 10a).

Histology
SPNs frequently undergo cystic degeneration and present as large hemorrhagic masses located in the pancreas. The tumor is arranged in solid or pseudopapillary architectural patterns and is admixed with hemorrhagic-necrotic foci of varying proportions. The tumor cells are monomorphic, poorly cohesive, and separated by hyalinized to myxoid stroma with thin-walled blood vessels. It is these blood vessels that give rise to the pseudopapillary appearance when the loosely cohesive tumor cells drop out, leaving tumor cells arranged around these fibrovascular stalks. True gland formation is not present. The tumor cells have a moderate amount of eosinophilic to clear cytoplasm. The nuclei have finely dispersed chromatin with nuclear grooves and indentations. Many intracellular and extracellular hyaline globules may be present (Fig. 10e).

Various studies have described histological criteria such as deep extrapancreatic extension, diffuse architecture, vascular invasion, peritoneal invasion, tumor necrosis, cellular pleomorphism and atypia, and increased mitotic activity [56, 57] to be associated with SPNs with aggressive clinical course. The proliferation marker Ki-67 is also said to be increased (usually 10% or more) in these cases [58]. However, none of these features have been confirmed as reliable markers of aggressiveness. The only morphological pattern associated with aggressive behavior found in one study was the presence of an undifferentiated component [59].

Cytology
The smears are cellular and are composed of monomorphic cells that are weakly adherent around the thin-walled blood vessels or may form pseudorosettes (Fig. 10b). The core of these papillary structures is formed of a capillary surrounded by variably thick, fibrous tissue with variable hyaliniza-

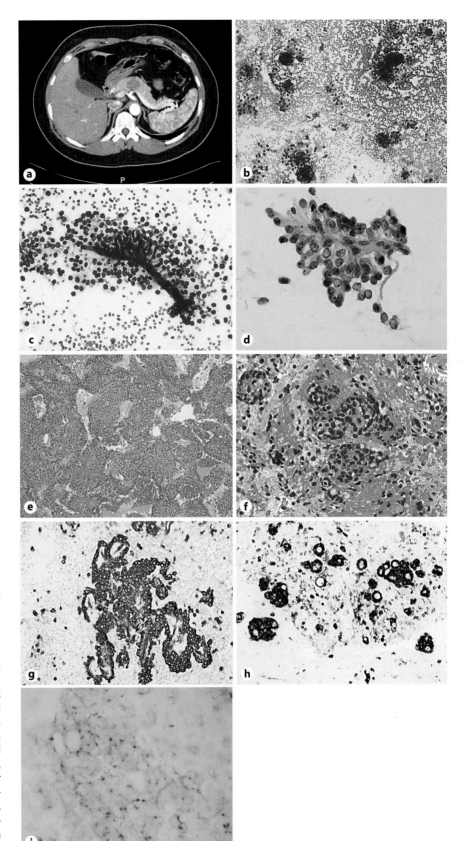

Fig. 10. SPN. **a** CT scan showing a hypodense neoplasm with smooth borders in the pancreatic head-body junction. **b** Monomorphic tumor cells with a moderate amount of cytoplasm and pseudorosette formation. Diff-Quik stain, ×10. **c** Tumor cells arranged loosely around a blood vessel, some exhibiting a long cytoplasmic processes. Diff-Quik stain, ×40. **d** Round to oval tumor cell nuclei with pale chromatin, nuclear indentations, and grooves. Papanicolaou stain, ×60. **e** Monomorphic tumor cells present around vessels and separated by hyalinized stroma. HE stain, ×10. **f** Cell block section with tumor cells forming pseudorosettes around hyalinized and myxoid stroma. HE stain, ×20. **g–i** Immunohistochemical stains. **g** Vimentin, ×20. **h** Nuclear β-catenin, ×20. **i** CD99 in a perinuclear dot-like pattern, ×40.

tion and myxoid changes. The cells are connected to the fibrovascular cores by wisps of cytoplasm (cytoplasmic "tails"), which are longest in the cells that are more distant from the fibrovascular cores (Fig. 10c) [60]. The background is composed of numerous bare nuclei with a stripped off cytoplasm, hemorrhage, foamy macrophages, and multinucleated giant cells. Individual tumor cells have a moderate amount of foamy to eosinophilic cytoplasm that may contain hyaline globules. The nucleus is round to oval and is frequently grooved and indented (Fig. 10d).

Key Cytological Features

- Low-power pattern described as spaghetti or Chinese letters
- Papillary fronds with a central fibrovascular core, middle layer of mucinous stroma, and outer layer of neoplastic cells
- Monomorphic cells with a scant to variable cytoplasm which may contain hyaline globules
- Round to oval nuclei, nuclear grooves, and indentations noted
- Tumor cells may show cytoplasmic "tails"
- Mucinous stroma is pathognomonic, and may be seen singly or surrounded by neoplastic cells

Ancillary Studies

SPNs uniformly show nuclear/cytoplasmic expression for β-catenin, due to mutation of the *CTNNB1* gene at exon 3 encoding this protein [61]. Lymphoid enhancing factor 1 (LEF1) and transcription factor for immunoglobulin heavy-chain enhancer 3 (TFE3), both in the Wnt/β-catenin signaling pathway, are also expressed in SPN and have been tested in cytology samples. An important caveat is that other neoplasms will have a similar expression for β-catenin, LEF1, and TFE3 if they harbor mutations in *CTNBB1*.

Loss of e-cadherin, or else nuclear localization of e-cadherin are also observed [62]. CD99 in a paranuclear dot-like expression is very specific for SPN, and is not identified in other non-ductal neoplasms [63]. Other markers that are strongly positive are vimentin, CD56, CD10, cyclin D1, progesterone receptor, androgen receptor, and alpha 1 antitrypsin. SPNs are usually negative for cytokeratins, although focal expression for CAM5.2 may be seen. Synaptophysin may be focally positive (Fig. 10f–i).

Differential Diagnosis

The differential diagnosis includes low-grade PanNETs and ACCs. Pathognomonic cytological features of SPNs, such as

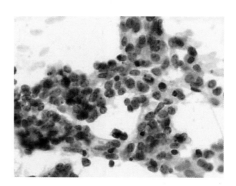

Fig. 11. Pancreatoblastoma. Elongated, columnar cells with abundant delicate cytoplasm with large, round basilar nuclei with prominent nucleoli from areas with acinar formations. Papanicolaou stain, ×40. Reproduced from Pitman and Faquin [69] with permission from John Wiley and Sons.

pseudorosettes with fibrotic stroma with hyalinized and myxoid change, tumor cells with cytoplasmic "tails," intracytoplasmic hyaline globules, and nuclear grooves, are helpful in distinguishing SPNs from other tumors. An immunohistochemical staining pattern that is positive for vimentin, CD99, and β-catenin (nuclear/cytoplasmic), and negative for trypsin and chymotrypsin support a diagnosis of SPN. PanNETs will express neuroendocrine markers and are negative for CD99. They retain e-cadherin and usually lack alterations in β-catenin staining.

Pancreatoblastoma

Pancreatoblastoma is defined by the WHO as an uncommon malignant epithelial neoplasm characterized by neoplastic cells with acinar differentiation and distinctive squamoid nests. Endocrine and ductal differentiation can occasionally occur [64].

Clinical Presentation

These tumors are one of the most common childhood pancreatic tumors with approximately a quarter of pancreatic tumors occurring in the first decade of life belonging to this category. Rare cases also occur in adults. Tumors associated with the Beckwith-Wiedemann syndrome are almost always cystic [65]. Common sites of metastases include liver, lymph nodes, and lung. Alpha-fetoprotein is elevated in many of these tumors. This serum marker is often used to follow patients for recurrent pancreatoblastoma. Many patients are asymptomatic and the tumor is discovered incidentally. Common presenting symptoms include abdominal pain,

Table 2. Comparison of salient features of PanNET, ACC, SPN, and pancreatoblastoma

Tumor	Age	Sex ratio	Associated syndromes	Gross features and location	Imaging findings	Cytological findings	Immunoprofile
PanNET	30–60 years	M:F 1:1	MEN1, tuberous sclerosis, VHL, neurofibromatosis	Solid, a few are cystic Commonly located in head of pancreas	Hypervascular well-circumscribed mass	Monomorphic epithelial cells, eccentric cytoplasm, salt and pepper chromatin	Positive for CK8 and 18, INSM1, synaptophysin, chromogranin
ACC	Adults 20–88 years 15% of cases in pediatric patients	M:F 2.1:1	Lynch syndrome, FAP	Solid, fleshy Cystic foci can be admixed Located anywhere in the pancreas but more common in the head	Large tumors, homogeneous, relatively well circumscribed	Minimally pleomorphic cells with moderate to abundant granular cytoplasm, prominent nucleoli, forming acini, numerous mitotic figures	Positive for trypsin, chymotrypsin, BCL10 Nuclear β-catenin in some cases
SPN	7–79 years	M:F 1:9	FAP	Large, round, fluctuant solitary masses with hemorrhage Located anywhere in the pancreas	Sharply demarcated heterogeneous mass without internal septations	Monomorphic epithelial cells loosely adherent around blood vessels, forming pseudorosettes, cells with cytoplasmic "tails," hyaline globules, and nuclear grooves and indentations	Positive for β-catenin (nuclear), CD10, CD99 (paranuclear dot-like pattern), AR, PR, vimentin Focal positivity for CAM5.2, synaptophysin
Pancreatoblastoma	Majority are pediatric patients Median age 4 years Few adults 18–78 years	M:F 1.3:1	Beckwith-Wiedemann syndrome	Large, solid, solitary tumors, Rarely cystic Located anywhere in the pancreas	Well-defined, heterogeneous masses with calcifications	Undifferentiated small cells, focal acinar differentiation and squamoid nests, primitive mesenchyme	Positive for CK7, CK8 and 18, CK19, and alpha-fetoprotein Squamoid morules positive for β-catenin (nuclear) Acinar cell foci positive for trypsin, chymotrypsin, BCL10 Neuroendocrine component positive for chromogranin, synaptophysin

PanNET, pancreatic neuroendocrine tumor; ACC, acinar cell carcinoma; SPN, solid pseudopapillary neoplasm; MEN1, multiple endocrine neoplasia 1; VHL, von Hippel-Lindau; FAP, familial adenomatous polyposis; CK, cytokeratin; AR, androgen receptor; PR, progesterone receptor.

nausea, diarrhea, and weight loss. Jaundice and gastrointestinal bleeding are other symptoms that are not very common.

Imaging
On radiographic examination, pancreatoblastomas appear as well-defined, heterogeneous masses that may be calcified.

Histology
Pancreatoblastomas are usually large at presentation, with a mean size of 11 cm [64]. The tumors are well circumscribed and fleshy. The foci of necrosis may be admixed. The tumors are very cellular and are arranged in well-defined nests that are separated by stromal bands. The tumor is composed of cells of varying differentiation ranging from small undifferentiated cells to cells with acinar differentiation and squamoid nests. Solid foci of undifferentiated tumor cells alternate with cells with acinar differentiation in

the form of cells arranged around central lumina with prominent nucleoli. Rare foci with gland-like structures or a neuroendocrine component may be present. A characteristic histologic finding in pancreatoblastoma is the presence of squamoid nests. These are foci of cells composed of whorled spindle cells with a squamous appearance or occasionally keratinizing squamous cells that are randomly scattered in the tumor. Pancreatoblastoma has a stromal component, Osseous or chondroid metaplasia may occasionally be seen [64].

Cytology
The smears are very cellular, composed of cells showing multilinear differentiation. The tumor cells are polygonal with round to oval nuclei. Small nucleoli may be present. The cytoplasm may be granular, eosinophilic to amphophilic, resembling acinar cells. The main cell type is a small, blast-like tumor cell with a high nuclear-to-cytoplasmic ra-

tio, fine immature chromatin, and small but distinctive nucleoli, present in clusters as well as singly (Fig. 11) [66]. On FNA smears the squamoid nests/morules appear as larger streaming or whorled cells with more abundant, squamoid-appearing cytoplasm [66]. The nuclear-to-cytoplasmic ratio is low, and they have elongated, oval nuclei with clear chromatin. They are more readily seen in cell block sections. The nuclei in squamoid nests may be optically clear. Cells with typical acinar or neuroendocrine morphological features are also seen.

The stromal components may also be appreciated on cytology. In a case reported by Zhu et al. [67], the aspirate is described as cellular containing biphasic components. The mesenchymal component was reported to be composed of primitive spindle-shaped cells associated with spiderweb-like intertwining long and fine fibrils. The epithelial component was described as sharp, angulated cohesive tissue fragments composed of medium-sized cells with an amphophilic cytoplasm. The tumor cells had a syncytial appearance due to indistinct cell borders.

Key Cytological Features
- Small blast-like cells, with a high nuclear-to-cytoplasmic ratio present singly and in clusters
- Biphasic tumor composed of primitive mesenchyme and undifferentiated epithelial cells
- Focal acinar cell differentiation
- Focal neuroendocrine differentiation
- Presence of squamoid nests/morules of cells

Ancillary Studies
Pancreatoblastomas express cytokeratins, including CK7, CK8, CK18, and CK19, and alpha-fetoprotein. Foci of acinar differentiation are positive for trypsin, chymotrypsin, and BCL10, and foci of neuroendocrine differentiation are positive for INSM1, synaptophysin, and chromogranin. The cells of squamous nests show nuclear/cytoplasmic expression for β-catenin, and this feature is useful for identifying them when they are subtle. The squamoid morules do not express the typical markers of squamous differentiation but instead express CK8, CK18, CK19, epithelial membrane antigen, and cyclin D1. There may be scattered positivity for CK 5/6 in the squamoid nests and other tumor cell types [68].

Differential Diagnosis
The differential diagnosis includes PanNET, ACC, mixed acinar-NEC, PDAC, and SPN. Cell block material is very helpful in making a diagnosis of pancreatoblastoma since the presence of squamoid corpuscles, a key element for diagnosing pancreatoblastoma, are better appreciated on the cell block material [69], although it can be recognized on smears [66]. The salient features of PanNET, ACC, SPN, and pancreatoblastomas are listed in Table 2.

Disclosure Statement

The author has no conflicts of interest to disclose.

References

1 Rindi G, Arnold R, Bosman F, Capella C, Klimstra D, Kloppel G, Komminoth P, Solcia E: Nomenclature and classification of neuroendocrine neoplasms of the digestive system; in Bosman F, Carneiro F, Hruban R, Theise N (eds): WHO Classification Tumours of the Digestive System, ed 4. Lyon, IARC Press, 2010, p 13.

2 Vagefi PA, Razo O, Deshpande V, McGrath DJ, Lauwers GY, Thayer SP, Warshaw AL, Fernandez-Del Castillo C: Evolving patterns in the detection and outcomes of pancreatic neuroendocrine neoplasms: the Massachusetts General Hospital experience from 1977 to 2005. Arch Surg 2007;142: 347–354.

3 Reid MD, Balci S, Saka B, Adsay NV: Neuroendocrine tumors of the pancreas: current concepts and controversies. Endocr Pathol 2014;25:65–79.

4 Shi C, Klimstra DS: Pancreatic neuroendocrine tumors: pathologic and molecular characteristics. Semin Diagn Pathol 2014;31:498–511.

5 Yachida S, Vakiani E, White CM, Zhong Y, Saunders T, Morgan R, de Wilde RF, Maitra A, Hicks J, Demarzo AM, Shi C, Sharma R, Laheru D, Edil BH, Wolfgang CL, Schulick RD, Hruban RH, Tang LH, Klimstra DS, Iacobuzio-Donahue CA: Small cell and large cell neuroendocrine carcinomas of the pancreas are genetically similar and distinct from well-differentiated pancreatic neuroendocrine tumors. Am J Surg Pathol 2012;36:173–184.

6 Sorbye H, Strosberg J, Baudin E, Klimstra DS, Yao JC: Gastroenteropancreatic high-grade neuroendocrine carcinoma. Cancer 2014;120:2814–2823.

7 Kloppel G, Couvelard A, Hruban RH, Klimstra DS, Komminoth P, osamura RY, Rindi G: Introduction; in Lloyd RV, Osamura RY, Kloppel G, Rosai J (eds): WHO Classification of Tumours of Neuroendocrine Origin. Lyon, IARC Press, 2017, pp 211–214.

8 Klimstra DS, Kloppel G, La Rosa S, Rindi G: Classification of neuroendocrine neoplasms of the digestive system; in WHO Classification of Tumours Editorial Board (eds): WHO Classification of Tumours, ed 5. Lyon, IARC Press, 2019, pp 16–19.

9 Reid MD, Bagci P, Ohike N, Saka B, Erbarut Seven I, Dursun N, Balci S, Gucer H, Jang KT, Tajiri T, Basturk O, Kong SY, Goodman M, Akkas G, Adsay V: Calculation of the Ki67 index in pancreatic neuroendocrine tumors: a comparative analysis of four counting methodologies. Mod Pathol 2015; 28:686–694.

10 Farrell JM, Pang JC, Kim GE, Tabatabai ZL: Pancreatic neuroendocrine tumors: accurate grading with Ki-67 index on fine-needle aspiration specimens using the WHO 2010/ENETS criteria. Cancer Cytopathol 2014;122:770–778.

11 Diaz Del Arco C, Esteban Lopez-Jamar JM, Ortega Medina L, Diaz Perez JA, Fernandez Acenero MJ: Fine-needle aspiration biopsy of pancreatic neuroendocrine tumors: correlation between Ki-67 index in cytological samples and clinical behavior. Diagn Cytopathol 2017;45:29–35.

12 Marchegiani G, Crippa S, Malleo G, Partelli S, Capelli P, Pederzoli P, Falconi M: Surgical treatment of pancreatic tumors in childhood and adolescence: uncommon neoplasms with favorable outcome. Pancreatology 2011;11:383–389.

13 Dial PF, Braasch JW, Rossi RL, Lee AK, Jin GL: Management of nonfunctioning islet cell tumors of the pancreas. Surg Clin North Am 1985;65: 291–299.

14 Venkatesh S, Ordonez NG, Ajani J, Schultz PN, Hickey RC, Johnston DA, Samaan NA: Islet cell carcinoma of the pancreas. A study of 98 patients. Cancer 1990;65:354–357.

15 Metz DC, Jensen RT: Gastrointestinal neuroendocrine tumors: pancreatic endocrine tumors. Gastroenterology 2008;135:1469–1492.

16 Kulke MH, Anthony LB, Bushnell DL, de Herder WW, Goldsmith SJ, Klimstra DS, Marx SJ, Pasieka JL, Pommier RF, Yao JC, Jensen RT; North American Neuroendocrine Tumor Society: NANETS treatment guidelines: well-differentiated neuroendocrine tumors of the stomach and pancreas. Pancreas 2010;39:735–752.

17 Service FJ: Insulinoma and other islet-cell tumors. Cancer Treat Res 1997;89:335–346.

18 Grozinsky-Glasberg S, Mazeh H, Gross DJ: Clinical features of pancreatic neuroendocrine tumors. J Hepatobiliary Pancreat Sci 2015;22:578–585.

19 Atiq M, Bhutani MS, Bektas M, Lee JE, Gong Y, Tamm EP, Shah CP, Ross WA, Yao J, Raju GS, Wang X, Lee JH: EUS-FNA for pancreatic neuroendocrine tumors: a tertiary cancer center experience. Dig Dis Sci 2012;57:791–800.

20 Lawrence B, Gustafsson BI, Kidd M, Pavel M, Svejda B, Modlin IM: The clinical relevance of chromogranin A as a biomarker for gastroenteropancreatic neuroendocrine tumors. Endocrinol Metab Clin North Am 2011;40:111–134.

21 Eriksson B, Oberg K, Stridsberg M: Tumor markers in neuroendocrine tumors. Digestion 2000; 62(suppl 1):33–38.

22 O'Dorisio TM, Krutzik SR, Woltering EA, Lindholm E, Joseph S, Gandolfi AE, Wang YZ, Boudreaux JP, Vinik AI, Go VL, Howe JR, Halfdanarson T, O'Dorisio MS, Mamikunian G: Development of a highly sensitive and specific carboxy-terminal human pancreastatin assay to monitor neuroendocrine tumor behavior. Pancreas 2010;39:611–616.

23 Dromain C, Deandreis D, Scoazec JY, Goere D, Ducreux M, Baudin E, Tselikas L: Imaging of neuroendocrine tumors of the pancreas. Diagn Interv Imaging 2016;97:1241–1257.

24 Fryer E, Serra S, Chetty R: Lipid-rich ("clear cell") neuroendocrine tumors of the pancreas in MEN I patients. Endocr Pathol 2012;23:243–246.

25 Chen S, Wang X, Lin J: Fine needle aspiration of oncocytic variants of pancreatic neuroendocrine tumor: a report of three misdiagnosed cases. Acta Cytol 2014;58:131–137.

26 Perez-Montiel MD, Frankel WL, Suster S: Neuroendocrine carcinomas of the pancreas with "rhabdoid" features. Am J Surg Pathol 2003;27:642–649.

27 Stokes MB, Kumar A, Symmans WF, Scholes JV, Melamed J: Pancreatic endocrine tumor with signet ring cell features: a case report with novel ultrastructural observations. Ultrastruct Pathol 1998;22:147–152.

28 Richmond AM, Mehrotra S: Two unusual variants of pancreatic neuroendocrine tumor and their potential pitfalls on fine-needle aspiration cytology. Diagn Cytopathol 2017;45:371–378.

29 Kaur G, Bakshi P, Singla V, Verma K: Clear cell neuroendocrine tumor of pancreas: endoscopic ultrasound-guided fine needle aspiration diagnosis of an uncommon variant. Cytojournal 2016;13: 7.

30 Safo AO, Li RW, Vickers SM, Schmechel SC, Pambuccian SE: Endoscopic ultrasound-guided fine-needle aspiration diagnosis of clear-cell pancreatic endocrine neoplasm in a patient with von Hippel-Lindau disease: a case report. Diagn Cytopathol 2009;37:365–372.

31 Singh R, Basturk O, Klimstra DS, Zamboni G, Chetty R, Hussain S, La Rosa S, Yilmaz A, Capelli P, Capella C, Cheng JD, Adsay NV: Lipid-rich variant of pancreatic endocrine neoplasms. Am J Surg Pathol 2006;30:194–200.

32 Fite JJ, Ali SZ, VandenBussche CJ: Fine-needle aspiration of a pancreatic neuroendocrine tumor with prominent rhabdoid features. Diagnostic Cytopathology 2018;46:600–603.

33 Tanigawa M, Nakayama M, Taira T, Hattori S, Mihara Y, Kondo R, Kusano H, Nakamura K, Abe Y, Ishida Y, Okabe Y, Hisaka T, Okuda K, Fujino K, Ito T, Kawahara A, Naito Y, Yamaguchi R, Akiba J, Akagi Y, Yano H: Insulinoma-associated protein 1 (INSM1) is a useful marker for pancreatic neuroendocrine tumor. Med Mol Morphol 2018; 51:32–40.

34 Ozcan A, Shen SS, Hamilton C, Anjana K, Coffey D, Krishnan B, Truong LD: PAX 8 expression in non-neoplastic tissues, primary tumors, and metastatic tumors: a comprehensive immunohistochemical study. Mod Pathol 2011;24:751–764.

35 Hermann G, Konukiewitz B, Schmitt A, Perren A, Kloppel G: Hormonally defined pancreatic and duodenal neuroendocrine tumors differ in their transcription factor signatures: expression of ISL1, PDX1, NGN3, and CDX2. Virchows Arch 2011;459:147–154.

36 Jiao Y, Shi C, Edil BH, de Wilde RF, Klimstra DS, Maitra A, Schulick RD, Tang LH, Wolfgang CL, Choti MA, Velculescu VE, Diaz LA Jr, Vogelstein B, Kinzler KW, Hruban RH, Papadopoulos N: DAXX/ATRX, MEN1, and mTOR pathway genes are frequently altered in pancreatic neuroendocrine tumors. Science 2011;331:1199–1203.

37 Kaemmerer D, Trager T, Hoffmeister M, Sipos B, Hommann M, Sanger J, Schulz S, Lupp A: Inverse expression of somatostatin and CXCR4 chemokine receptors in gastroenteropancreatic neuroendocrine neoplasms of different malignancy. Oncotarget 2015;6:27566–27579.

38 Sigel C, Reidy-Lagunes D, Lin O, Basturk O, Aggarwal G, Klimstra DS, Tang L: Cytological features contributing to the misclassification of pancreatic neuroendocrine tumors. J Am Soc Cytopathol 2016;5:266–276.

39 Tang LH, Basturk O, Sue JJ, Klimstra DS: A practical approach to the classification of WHO grade 3 (G3) well-differentiated neuroendocrine tumor (WD-NET) and poorly differentiated neuroendocrine carcinoma (PD-NEC) of the pancreas. Am J Surg Pathol 2016;40:1192–1202.

40 Konukiewitz B, Schlitter AM, Jesinghaus M, Pfister D, Steiger K, Segler A, Agaimy A, Sipos B, Zamboni G, Weichert W, Esposito I, Pfarr N, Kloppel G: Somatostatin receptor expression related to TP53 and RB1 alterations in pancreatic and extrapancreatic neuroendocrine neoplasms with a Ki67-index above 20. Mod Pathol 2017;30: 587–598.

41 La Rosa S, Klimstra DS, Wood LD: Pancreatic acinar cell carcinoma; in WHO Classification of Tumours Editorial Board (ed): Digestive System Tumours, ed 5. Lyon, IARC Press, 2019, pp 333–336.

42 Seth AK, Argani P, Campbell KA, Cameron JL, Pawlik TM, Schulick RD, Choti MA, Wolfgang CL: Acinar cell carcinoma of the pancreas: an institutional series of resected patients and review of the current literature. J Gastrointest Surg 2008;12: 1061–1067.

43 Kuerer H, Shim H, Pertsemlidis D, Unger P: Functioning pancreatic acinar cell carcinoma: immunohistochemical and ultrastructural analyses. Am J Clin Oncol 1997;20:101–107.

44 Sigel CS, Klimstra DS: Cytomorphologic and immunophenotypical features of acinar cell neoplasms of the pancreas. Cancer Cytopathol 2013; 121:459–470.

45 Labate AM, Klimstra DL, Zakowski MF: Comparative cytologic features of pancreatic acinar cell carcinoma and islet cell tumor. Diagn Cytopathol 1997;16:112–116.

46 Ordonez NG: Pancreatic acinar cell carcinoma. Adv Anat Pathol 2001;8:144–159.

47 La Rosa S, Franzi F, Marchet S, Finzi G, Clerici M, Vigetti D, Chiaravalli AM, Sessa F, Capella C: The monoclonal anti-BCL10 antibody (clone 331.1) is a sensitive and specific marker of pancreatic acinar cell carcinoma and pancreatic metaplasia. Virchows Arch 2009;454:133–142.

48 Hoorens A, Lemoine NR, McLellan E, Morohoshi T, Kamisawa T, Heitz PU, Stamm B, Ruschoff J, Wiedenmann B, Kloppel G: Pancreatic acinar cell carcinoma. An analysis of cell lineage markers, p53 expression, and Ki-ras mutation. Am J Pathol 1993;143:685–698.

49 Ohike N, Kosmahl M, Kloppel G: Mixed acinar-endocrine carcinoma of the pancreas. A clinicopathological study and comparison with acinar-cell carcinoma. Virchows Arch 2004;445:231–235.

50 La Rosa S, Sessa F, Capella C: Acinar cell carcinoma of the pancreas: overview of clinicopathologic features and insights into the molecular pathology. Front Med 2015;2:41.

51 Klimstra DS, Rosai J, Heffess CS: Mixed acinar-endocrine carcinomas of the pancreas. Am J Surg Pathol 1994;18:765–778.

52 Kloppel G, Basturk O, Klimstra DS, Lam AK, Notohara K: Solid pseudopappilary neoplasm of the pancreas; in WHO Classification of Tumours Editorial Board (ed): Digestive System Tumours, ed 5. Lyon, IARC Press, 2019, pp 340–342.

53 Papavramidis T, Papavramidis S: Solid pseudopapillary tumors of the pancreas: review of 718 patients reported in English literature. J Am Coll Surg 2005;200:965–972.

54 Kang CM, Kim KS, Choi JS, Kim H, Lee WJ, Kim BR: Solid pseudopapillary tumor of the pancreas suggesting malignant potential. Pancreas 2006;32: 276–280.

55 Klimstra DS, Wenig BM, Heffess CS: Solid-pseudopapillary tumor of the pancreas: a typically cystic carcinoma of low malignant potential. Semin Diagn Pathol 2000;17:66–80.

56 Matsunou H, Konishi F: Papillary-cystic neoplasm of the pancreas. A clinicopathologic study concerning the tumor aging and malignancy of nine cases. Cancer 1990;65:283–291.

57 Nishihara K, Nagoshi M, Tsuneyoshi M, Yamaguchi K, Hayashi I: Papillary cystic tumors of the pancreas. Assessment of their malignant potential. Cancer 1993;71:82–92.

58 Watanabe Y, Okamoto K, Okada K, Aikawa M, Koyama I, Yamaguchi H: A case of aggressive solid pseudopapillary neoplasm: comparison of clinical and pathologic features with non-aggressive cases. Pathol Int 2017;67:202–207.

59 Tang LH, Aydin H, Brennan MF, Klimstra DS: Clinically aggressive solid pseudopapillary tumors of the pancreas: a report of two cases with components of undifferentiated carcinoma and a comparative clinicopathologic analysis of 34 conventional cases. Am J Surg Pathol 2005;29:512–519.

60 Samad A, Shah AA, Stelow EB, Alsharif M, Cameron SE, Pambuccian SE: Cercariform cells: another cytologic feature distinguishing solid pseudopapillary neoplasms from pancreatic endocrine neoplasms and acinar cell carcinomas in endoscopic ultrasound-guided fine-needle aspirates. Cancer Cytopathol 2013;121:298–310.

61 Tanaka Y, Kato K, Notohara K, Hojo H, Ijiri R, Miyake T, Nagahara N, Sasaki F, Kitagawa N, Nakatani Y, Kobayashi Y: Frequent beta-catenin mutation and cytoplasmic/nuclear accumulation in pancreatic solid-pseudopapillary neoplasm. Cancer Res 2001;61:8401–8404.

62 Serra S, Chetty R: Revision 2: an immunohistochemical approach and evaluation of solid pseudopapillary tumour of the pancreas. J Clin Pathol 2008;61:1153–1159.

63 Guo Y, Yuan F, Deng H, Wang HF, Jin XL, Xiao JC: Paranuclear dot-like immunostaining for CD99: a unique staining pattern for diagnosing solid-pseudopapillary neoplasm of the pancreas. Am J Surg Pathol 2011;35:799–806.

64 Ohike N, La Rosa S: Pancreatoblastoma; in WHO Classification of Tumours Editorial Board (eds): Digestive System Tumors. WHO Classification of Tumors, ed 5. Lyon, IARC Press, 2019, pp 337–339.

65 Drut R, Jones MC: Congenital pancreatoblastoma in Beckwith-Wiedemann syndrome: an emerging association. Pediatr Pathol 1988;8:331–339.

66 Reid MD, Bhattarai S, Graham RP, Pehlivanoglu B, Sigel CS, Shi J, Saqi A, Shirazi M, Xue Y, Basturk O, Adsay V: Pancreatoblastoma: cytologic and histologic analysis of 12 adult cases reveals helpful criteria in their diagnosis and distinction from common mimics. Cancer Cytopathol 2019; 127:708–719.

67 Zhu LC, Sidhu GS, Cassai ND, Yang GC: Fine-needle aspiration cytology of pancreatoblastoma in a young woman: report of a case and review of the literature. Diagn Cytopathol 2005;33:258–262.

68 Nishimata S, Kato K, Tanaka M, Ijiri R, Toyoda Y, Kigasawa H, Ohama Y, Nakatani Y, Notohara K, Kobayashi Y, Horie H, Hoshika A, Tanaka Y: Expression pattern of keratin subclasses in pancreatoblastoma with special emphasis on squamoid corpuscles. Pathol Int 2005;55:297–302.

69 Pitman MB, Faquin WC: The fine-needle aspiration biopsy cytology of pancreatoblastoma. Diagn Cytopathol 2004;31:402–406.

Jasreman Dhillon, MD
Moffitt Cancer Center
12902 USF Magnolia Drive
Tampa, FL 33612 (USA)
jasreman.dhillon@moffitt.org

Chapter 9

Published online: September 29, 2020

Centeno BA, Dhillon J (eds): Pancreatic Tumors. Monogr Clin Cytol. Basel, Karger, 2020, vol 26, pp 109–121
(DOI:10.1159/000455738)

Metastases, Secondary Tumors, and Lymphomas of the Pancreas

Barbara A. Centeno[a, b]

[a]Department of Pathology, Moffitt Cancer Center, Tampa, FL, USA; [b]Department of Oncologic Sciences, University of South Florida Morsani College of Medicine, Tampa, FL, USA

Abstract

The pancreas is infrequently the site of secondary involvement by solid or hematopoietic malignancies. While carcinomas and melanoma are the most common malignancies to secondarily involve the pancreas, the literature is replete with reports of uncommon and rare entities metastasizing to the pancreas. Fine-needle aspiration is indicated to establish the diagnosis and direct patient management. Diagnostic accuracy depends on correlation with clinical and imaging findings, previous pathology if known, and selection of the appropriate ancillary studies. Here we review the cytopathology of secondary tumors involving the pancreas and provide an approach to the diagnostic work-up. © 2020 S. Karger AG, Basel

The antemortem detection of secondary malignancies of the pancreas has increased significantly over the last 3 decades due to improvements of imaging, utilization of serum markers for the surveillance of malignancy, and the use of fine-needle aspiration (FNA). The most common metastases encountered in autopsy studies are lung (25%), breast (13%), melanoma (11%), stomach (10%), colorectal (6%), kidney (4%), ovary (4%), and others (27%) [1]. In earlier clinical series, lung primaries remained the most common, but kidney primaries were the second most common. The average distribution was lung (23%), kidney (15%), breast (8%), colorectal (8%), melanoma (5%), liver (5%), and others (36%) [1]. In more recent clinical series focused on preoperative diagnosis with FNA and small biopsies, renal cell carcinoma was the most common [2].

Neoplasms originating outside of the pancreas may involve the pancreas by direct extension, through hematogenous or lymphatic metastases, or as a manifestation of systemic disease as with lymphomas and leukemias [1]. Malignancies involving the pancreas by direct extension most often originate from adjacent organs or organs in close proximity such as the stomach, duodenum, colon, and gallbladder [3].

Clinical and Imaging Presentation

Pancreatic metastases are detected either at the time of initial diagnosis during the work-up for metastasis, during surveillance for an established primary, or with symptoms due to the metastases [3]. Pancreatic metastases are most commonly detected when patients undergo surveillance imaging for a known primary malignancy, and most patients are asymptomatic, in contrast to patients with primary pancreatic ductal adenocarcinoma (PDAC), who are more often symptomatic [4–6]. Presenting symptoms are non-specific and include abdominal pain, gastrointestinal bleeding, and weight loss. Some patients may present with obstruction of the common biliary duct (CBD) with jaundice and obstruction of the main pancreatic duct (MPD) and acute pancreatitis, although MPD and CBD obstruction with jaundice are less frequently encountered in metastases compared to PDAC [5, 7, 8].

Computed tomographic imaging shows three main patterns of tissue involvement: solitary (50–73%), multiple (5–19%), and diffusely infiltrative (15–44%) [4]. Breast and small-cell carcinoma more commonly present as diffusely infiltrative lesions. Lesions may be homogenous, heterogeneous, or peripherally enhancing with a hypodense focus due to tumor necrosis. The tumors may be round, ovoid, and well circumscribed, or else ill defined with an infiltrative margin. The majority are solid, but some may be cystic or have a cystic component. They may be isodense or hypodense, and hypovascular or hypervascular. These imaging patterns overlap with primary pancreatic malignancies and neoplasms and may lead to an erroneous diagnosis of a new pancreatic primary if the patient does not have an established history of malignancy.

Special consideration will be given to the imaging findings of renal cell carcinoma, since it is the most frequently encountered metastasis in the most recent FNA series. Renal cell carcinoma tends to metastasize as a solitary lesion to the pancreas, many years after the original diagnosis. On imaging, it is hypodense and hypervascular, similar to pancreatic neuroendocrine tumor (PanNET). Adding to the difficulty in the differential diagnosis with PanNET is that renal cell carcinoma expresses somatostatin receptors, and therefore they will be detected with Octreoscan scintigraphy [9]. Patients with von-Hippel Lindau (VHL) syndrome are at risk of developing both renal cell carcinoma and PanNET. In patients with a history of renal cell carcinoma and a new pancreatic mass, the potential of a new PanNET should be considered.

Cytological Diagnosis of Pancreatic Metastases

The first series describing the FNA diagnosis of pancreatic metastases was published by Benning et al. [10] in 1992. Nineteen out of 176 (10.8%) malignancies identified from 304 aspirates showed secondary involvement of the pancreas, including 7 non-Hodgkin's lymphoma, 2 Hodgkin's lymphomas, 3 small-cell carcinomas, 3 squamous cell carci-

nomas (2 cervix, 1 esophagus), and 1 hepatocellular carcinoma. Metastatic disease to the pancreas was the initial presentation in 6 of the 19 (32%) patients. The lymphomas and Hodgkin's lymphoma were theorized to have presented in the peripancreatic lymph nodes. Carson et al. [11] published their series in 1995, and 13 of 117 radiologically guided FNAs (11%) showed metastatic disease. Nine of 13 (69%) patients had a prior history of malignancy, while the other 4 (31%) presented with a pancreatic mass and were subsequently found to have widely metastatic disease. Fritscher-Ravens et al. [12] published the first series on EUS-FNA of pancreatic metastases. Twelve of the 114 (12.7%) patients studied had metastatic disease. Six of the 12 had a prior diagnosis of malignancy (3 breast, 2 renal cell, 1 salivary gland), and 6 did not have a prior history of malignancy (1 renal cell carcinoma, 1 colonic, 1 ovary, and 1 esophagus). One patient had an unknown primary, and another had a lymphoma.

Since this initial series on EUS-FNA for the diagnosis of pancreatic metastases, there have been a number of series describing the experience of FNA and small biopsies for the diagnosis of secondary malignancies in the pancreas [2, 7, 8, 13–27]. Raymond et al. [2] summarized their own experience with EUS-FNA, transabdominal FNA, and core-needle biopsies, and reviewed the published series from 1992 to 2016. Three additional series have since been published, 1 in 2017 [23], 1 in 2018 [27], and 1 in the Spanish language literature in 2019 [16]. Table 1 summarizes these studies. The study durations were from 2 to 26 years, and included between 112 and 5,495 total FNA or core-needle biopsy samples [2, 16, 23, 27]. The smallest case series consisted of 11 cases [21] and the largest consisted of 66 [26]. Pancreatic metastases accounted for 0.7–11.1% of all FNA and core-needle biopsies [2, 16, 23], and for 1.8–10.8% of all neoplasms [2, 16, 23, 27]. The majority of patients had their metastases detected during surveillance, but some were symptomatic. Symptoms included abdominal pain, jaundice, weight loss, and nausea and vomiting.

A key observation from these series is that the pancreatic metastasis was the initial diagnosis of malignancy in a number of patients, with a range from 0 to 50%. In the series by Waters et al. [26], all patients had a prior diagnosis. The authors noted that the study was performed in a cancer center, which could account for the fact that all patients had a prior diagnosis of malignancy. In the series by Fritscher-Ravens et al. [12], 50% of their patients had no prior diagnosis of malignancy. Pathologists should keep this observation in mind when reviewing pancreatic FNAs and consider the possibil-

Table 1. Clinical characteristics of FNA series

Study	Year	Study length, years	Total cases (FNA/CNB), n	Total cancers, n	Total metastases, n	% of total FNA/CNB	% of total malignancies	Age range, years (average)	Gender M:F
Benning [10]	1992	NA	304	176	19	6.3	10.8	47–79 (66)	9:10
Carson [11]	1995	8	117	NA	13	11.1	NA	38–81 (65)	10:3
Fritscher-Ravens [12]	2001	2	112	NA	12	10.7	NA	34–78 (61)	8:12
Mesa [21]	2004	3	468	191	11	2.4	5.8	NA	NA
Volmar [25]	2004	5	1,050	503	20	1.9	4.0	40–83 (61)	11:9
De Witt [17]	2005	6	NA	NA	24	NA	NA	33–83 (60)	15:9
Gilbert [19]	2011	5	1,172	NA	25	2.1	NA	40–80 (61)	11:14
Hijioka [7]	2011	14	NA	NA	28	NA	NA	32–78 (60)	13:15
Layfield [20]	2012	8	2,318	222	17	0.7	7.7	15–80 (61)	14:3
Ardengh [14]	2013	14	NA	NA	32	NA	NA	26–84 (60)	
Atiq [15]	2013	5	674	NA	23	3.4	NA	(64)	10:13
El Hajj [18]	2013	12	NA	NA	49	NA	NA	30–83 (63)	23:26
Olson [22]	2013	26	5,495	2,389	42	0.8	1.8	median 59	23:19
Waters [26]	2014	10	NA	1,406	66	NA	4.7	40–89 (63)	38:28
Smith [24]	2015	14	2,327	NA	22	0.9	NA	59–83 (71)	13:9
Alomari [13]	2016	7	1,346	NA	31	2.3	NA	49–86 (66)	19:12
Raymond [2]	2017	15	636	221	16	2.5	7.2	43–82 (62)	11:5
Sekulic [23]	2017	10	1137	594	25	2.2	4.2	53–71 (64)	13:13
Hou [27]	2018	8	NA	NA	30	NA	NA	25–82 (65.5)	18:12
Betes [16]	2019	12	1,128	NA	44	NA	NA	median 58.6	28:16

FNA, fine-needle aspiration; CNB, core-needle biopsy; NA, not available.

ity of a metastasis if the morphology is unusual or if imaging studies show evidence of disease outside of the pancreas.

The latency periods are variable. Some metastases were detected synchronously with the initial detection of malignancy, and some many years later. Renal cell carcinoma is notorious for presenting many years after the initial diagnosis. The mean interval is 10 years [28]. The longest latency that this author has identified is 36 years [27]. Lung cancer metastases present earlier, usually within the first 2 years. Melanoma and breast cancer usually present within 7 years, and colon cancer at the 2- to 3-year interval [29]. Betes et al. [16] summarized the latency periods of the cancers in their series. Lung cancer was the most frequently detected synchronously with the primary or else within 1 year after the primary diagnosis. Melanoma, gynecological, and colon primaries were the most frequent in the 1- to 5-year interval. Renal cell carcinoma was the most frequent at an interval greater than 5 years. The latency period from the diagnosis of the primary to presentation of the pancreatic mass should also be a consideration when assessing for primary versus metastatic disease.

Renal cell carcinoma is the most frequently reported metastatic malignancy to the pancreas in FNA series, and lung cancer is the second most frequent [2, 7, 8, 13–27]. The top 5 primary sites are kidney (renal cell carcinoma), lung (small-cell carcinoma and adenocarcinoma), skin (melanoma), gastrointestinal tract (colon), and gynecological (serous ovarian). Table 2 summarizes the distribution of primary sites for each study [2, 7, 8, 13–27].

Cytology and Ancillary Studies of Pancreatic Metastases from Solid Tumors

Metastatic malignancies retain the cytomorphological and immunophenotypical features of the primary site. The metastasis may appear somewhat different morphologically due to tumor heterogeneity. The cytological features of the most common metastases and the differential diagnosis will be discussed in this section.

Table 2. Site of origin of metastases showing the top 6 and uncommon types

Study	% kidney	% lung	% GI	% skin	% breast	% gyn	Uncommon types reported (n)
Benning [10]	0	21	16	5	0	11	NHL (7), Hodgkin's lymphoma (2), gallbladder (1), HCC (1)
Carson [11]	8	8	23	0	8	8	HCC (1), plasmacytoma (1), NHL (1), malignant phyllodes tumor (1), prostate (1)
Fritscher-Ravens [12]	25	8	25	0	17	8	NHL (1), unknown primary (1)
Mesa [21]	9	36	9	0	18	18	Uterine leiomyosarcoma (1), NHL (1)
Volmar [25]	45	15	10	15	10	10	Prostate (1), GIST (1)
De Witt [17]	42	17	13	25	0	0	HCC (1), leiomyosarcoma (1)
Gilbert [19]	52	16	4	12	4	4	Renal leiomyosarcoma (1), prostate (1), NET, extrapancreatic (1)
Hijioka [7]	25	21	14	7	7	11	
Layfield [20]	47	12	6	0	0	6	Medullary thyroid carcinoma (1), NHL (1), alveolar rhabdomyosarcoma (1)
Ardengh [14]	13	9	22	3	6	3	Mesothelioma (1), HCC (1), leiomyosarcoma (1), rhabdomyosarcoma (1)
Atiq [15]	17	22	17	13	0	9	NHL (4), adrenal (1), vagina (1)
El Hajj [18]	43	16	16	12	6	4	Urothelial (1), HCC (1), leiomyosarcoma (1)
Olson [22]	38	14	2	19	5	5	Solitary fibrous tumor (2), fibrolamellar HCC (1), pleomorphic sarcoma (1), MPNST (1), GIST (1), papillary thyroid carcinoma (1)
Waters [26]	39	14	9	9	9	6	Medullary thyroid carcinoma (1), prostate (1), appendix (1), synovial sarcoma (1), adrenal (2), liver (2), leiomyosarcoma (2)
Smith [24]	64	5	9	0	0	14	Urothelial (1), papillary thyroid carcinoma (1) prostate (1), mesenchymal chondrosarcoma (1)
Alomari [13]	26	23	10	3	6	6	DLBCL (2), plasmacytoma (2), urothelial (1) liposarcoma (1), chondrosarcoma (1), synovial sarcoma (1)
Raymond [2]	19	38	19	13	0	0	Olfactory neuroblastoma (1)
Sekulic [23]	40	8	5	0	1	4	Leiomyosarcoma (1); oral SqCC (1), maxillary sinus melanoma (1)
Hou [27]	36.7	16.7	6.7	10	6.7	3.3	Eye melanoma (1), liposarcoma (1), leiomyosarcoma (1), sarcoma, NOS (1), unknown primary (2)
Betes [16]	27.2	22.7	11.3	6	0	6	Sarcomas (2), plasmacytoma (1)

CNB, core-needle biopsy; DLBCL, diffuse large B-cell lymphoma; FNA, fine-needle aspiration; GI, gastrointestinal; GIST, GI stromal tumor; gyn, gynecological; HCC, hepatocellular carcinoma; MPNST, malignant peripheral nerve sheath tumor; NA, not available; NHL, non-Hodgkin's lymphoma; SqCC, squamous cell carcinoma.

Renal Cell Carcinoma

The conventional clear cell variant is the most frequently encountered. FNAs may be hemodiluted due the vascularity of these neoplasms. [30] Smears are composed of variably sized cells with a low nuclear-to-cytoplasmic ratio (Fig. 1a–c). The cells are arranged in sheets and clusters, or else singly. Cells may be centered on fibrovascular cores. The cytoplasm may be wispy, granular, or vacuolated, or a mixture. The nuclei are centrally or eccentrically placed. The cells may be associated with vascular fragments. The degree of nuclear atypia depends on the grade of the carcinoma. The nuclei range from slightly irregular nuclear membranes with nucleoli only discernible at high power to high-grade tumors with increasingly irregular nuclear membranes, prominent nucleoli visualized at ×100, and increased pleomorphism. The carcinoma is grade 4 according to the ISUP grading classification if the nuclear atypia is in the form of a multilobulated pleomorphic sarcomatoid component or rhabdoid component [30].

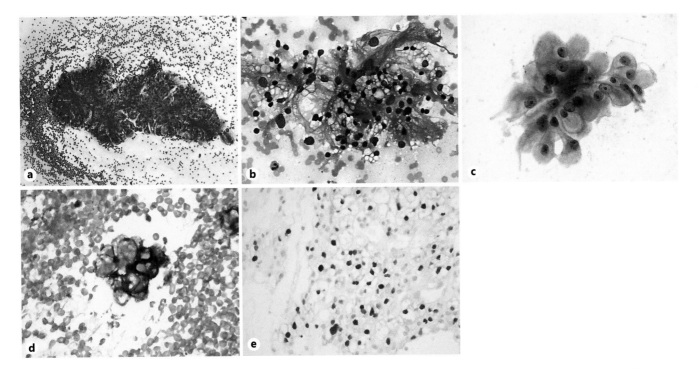

Fig. 1. Renal cell carcinoma. **a** Cohesive fragment of neoplastic cells with abundant cytoplasm, centered on a capillary framework. The background is hemorrhagic. Diff-Quik stain. **b** Cells with punched out vacuoles in the cytoplasm attached to a small vessel. Diff-Quik stain. **c** Cells with abundant, well-defined, clear cytoplasm. The nuclei are round with prominent nucleoli. **d** CD10 is strongly positive in the cytoplasm. Cell block, immunoperoxidase stain. **e** PAX8 is strongly positive in the nuclei. Cell block, immunoperoxidase stain.

Key Cytological Features
- Hemodiluted samples and bloody smears
- Papillary clusters, small groups, or single cells
- Small blood vessels
- Abundant cytoplasm with vacuoles
- Nuclear atypia depends on grade, nucleoli more prominent with increasing grade

Ancillary Studies
Clear cell renal cell carcinomas express PAX8 (Fig. 1d), CD10 (Fig. 1e), carbonic anhydrase IX (CA IX) (membranous pattern), vimentin, and renal cell antigen.

Differential Diagnosis
While the cytomorphology of clear cell renal cell carcinoma is distinct, the morphology may overlap with ductal adenocarcinomas with clear cell patterns. Ductal adenocarcinoma with a clear cell pattern forms nests or single cells with abundant, clear microvacuolated cytoplasm, a low nuclear-to-cytoplasmic ratio, and small nuclei with minimal nuclear membrane irregularities (Fig. 2a, b). A separate component

of the usual adenocarcinoma is usually present and will assist with the differential diagnosis.

Patients with von Hippel Lindau (VHL) syndrome are at risk of developing both renal cell carcinoma and PanNET. In patients with VHL and a history of renal cell carcinoma presenting with a new solitary pancreatic mass, the differential diagnosis includes PanNET. The PanNET occurring in these patients is usually the clear cell type. Diagnostic clues will be the presence of cells with a more typical plasmacytoid appearance or wispy, granular cytoplasm in addition to the clear cells. The nuclei retain the features typically described for PanNET, including monotonous nuclei, with round to oval, uniform nuclear membranes, and salt and pepper chromatin. PanNET will be positive for neuroendocrine markers, which will differentiate it from renal cell carcinoma.

Lung Cancer
Lung cancer is the next most frequently encountered metastasis in the pancreas. Small cell carcinoma (Fig. 3) is the most frequent type, followed by adenocarcinoma (Fig. 4a–c),

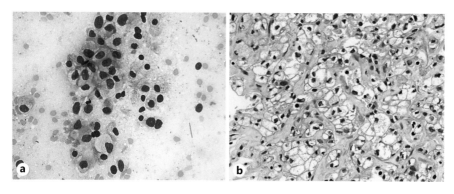

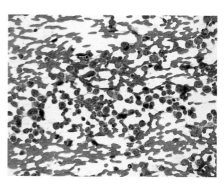

Fig. 2. PDAC with a clear cytoplasm. **a** The cytoplasm is well defined, and finely vacuolated. The nuclei are elongated or irregular, and lack prominent nucleoli. Diff-Quik stain. **b** Cell block showing adenocarcinoma with clear cytoplasm invading stroma. The carcinoma grows in small irregular groups. The nuclei are atypical and some are raisinoid. Cell block, HE stain.

Fig. 3. Pulmonary small-cell carcinoma. Small cells with scant cytoplasm, fusiform nuclei, fine, powdery chromatin, and focal molding. Papanicolaou stain.

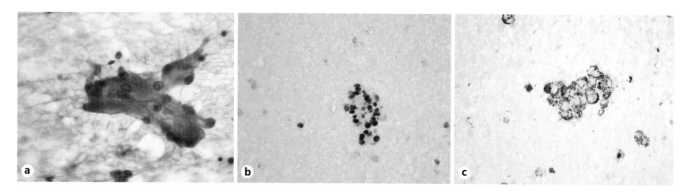

Fig. 4. Metastatic pulmonary adenocarcinoma. **a** Cells with well-defined cytoplasm containing mucin, enlarged nuclei. Papanicolaou stain. **b** TTF1 is strongly positive in the nuclei. Cell block, immunoperoxidase. **c** Napsin shows granular cytoplasmic expression. Cell block, immunoperoxidase.

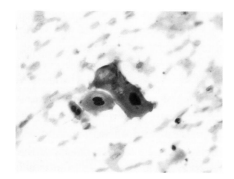

Fig. 5. Squamous cell carcinoma. Single, keratinized cells with smudgy, hyperchromatic chromatin. Papanicolaou stain.

squamous cell carcinoma (Fig. 5), and adenosquamous carcinomas.

Key Cytological Findings
• Depends on the subtype, variable

Ancillary Studies
Lung adenocarcinomas are positive for CK7, TTF1, and napsin (Fig. 4b, c).

Differential Diagnosis
The most difficult metastases to differentiate from a primary PDAC are pulmonary adenocarcinoma or adenosquamous carcinomas. Pancreatic carcinomas do not express TTF1 and napsin [31, 32], so these immunohistochemical markers are useful to diagnose a metastatic pulmonary non-

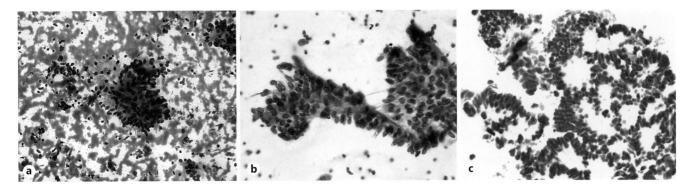

Fig. 6. Colonic adenocarcinoma. **a** Cigar-shaped cells in an acinar formation with feathering and background necrotic debris. Diff-Quik stain. **b** Columnar cells with elongated, cigar-shaped nuclei. Papanicolaou stain. **c** CDX2 is strongly positive in the nuclei. Cell block, immunoperoxidase stain.

small-cell carcinoma to the pancreas. This panel is not helpful when the morphology is that of a small-cell carcinoma, since extrapulmonary small-cell carcinomas express TTF1 [33].

Primary squamous cell carcinoma of the pancreas is exceedingly rare. Primary pancreatic small-cell carcinoma occurs but is less common than its pulmonary counterpart. Metastasis should always be considered in the setting of squamous cell or small-cell carcinoma involving the pancreas.

Gastrointestinal Adenocarcinomas
Colonic adenocarcinoma is the most common metastasis from the gastrointestinal tract. A smear showing an adenocarcinoma with elongated, cigar-shaped nuclei and abundant background necrosis may suggest a colorectal primary (Fig. 6a, b).

Key Cytological Findings
- Abundant background necrosis
- Columnar cells with cigar-shaped nuclei

Ancillary Studies
Colonic carcinomas are positive for CK20, CDX2 (Fig. 6c), MUC2, and Special AT-rich sequence-binding protein 2 (SATB2) , and negative for CK7 [34].

Differential Diagnosis
Metastatic colonic colloid carcinoma is more challenging (Fig. 7) as it overlaps morphologically and phenotypically with primary pancreatic colloid carcinoma. Both express CDX2. Colloid carcinoma of the pancreas develops from intraductal papillary mucinous carcinoma with an intestinal phenotype [35]. Correlation of the morphology with the imaging findings

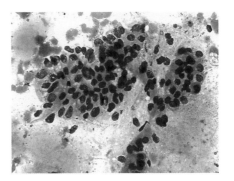

Fig. 7. Colonic colloid carcinoma with abundant background mucin and cytoplasmic mucin. Diff-Quik stain.

will be helpful, as the presence of a lesion suggestive of intraductal papillary mucinous neoplasm in the pancreas will point towards a primary colloid carcinoma. Esophageal and gastric primaries are more difficult to differentiate from pancreatic primaries as they have significant overlap in cytomorphological and immunophenotypic features.

Breast Carcinoma
Breast carcinomas are a frequent source of secondary tumors in the pancreas. The cytomorphology may be characteristic if the cells occur singly, with eccentric nuclei and cytoplasmic vacuoles (Fig. 8a, b). A high-grade breast carcinoma will be difficult to differentiate morphologically from PDAC.

Key Cytological Findings
- Dyshesive single cells
- Eccentric nuclei, targetoid cytoplasmic vacuoles

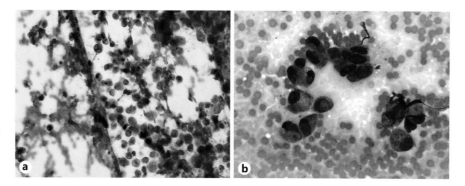

Fig. 8. Metastatic breast carcinoma. **a** Dyshesive cell population. The cells have eccentrically placed nuclei. Papanicolaou stain. **b** Single cells with eccentric nuclei, cytoplasmic vacuoles, and small, cytoplasmic, targetoid vacuoles. Diff-Quik stain.

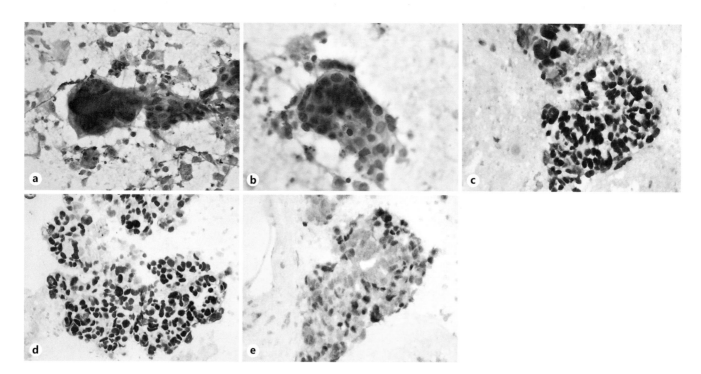

Fig. 9. Ovarian serous primary. **a** Carcinoma with pleomorphic, multinucleated malignant cells and a small sheet of malignant cells. Papanicolaou stain. **b** Papillary cluster. Papanicolaou stain. **c** PAX8. **d** p53. **e** WT1 are strongly expressed in the nuclei. Cell block, immunoperoxidase stain.

Ancillary Studies

Breast cancer expresses GATA3, gross cystic disease fluid protein-15 (GCDFP-15 or BRST2), and mammaglobin. Estrogen receptor and progesterone receptor are useful to identify breast as the site of origin, if the carcinoma expresses them.

Differential Diagnosis

Breast cancers express GATA3, but PDAC may also express GATA3 [36]. The breast markers mammaglobin and GCDFP-15 may be helpful. If the primary cancer was positive for estrogen receptor and progesterone receptor, it will be of added value to use these markers.

Gynecological Primaries

Gynecological primaries were the fifth most frequent primary sites encountered in the series, and ovarian serous primaries were the most common. These are characterized by pleomorphic malignant cells with abundant cytoplasm. The cells may form papillae (Fig. 9a, b). Endometrial adenocarcinomas and cervical squamous cell carcinomas are also reported in these series.

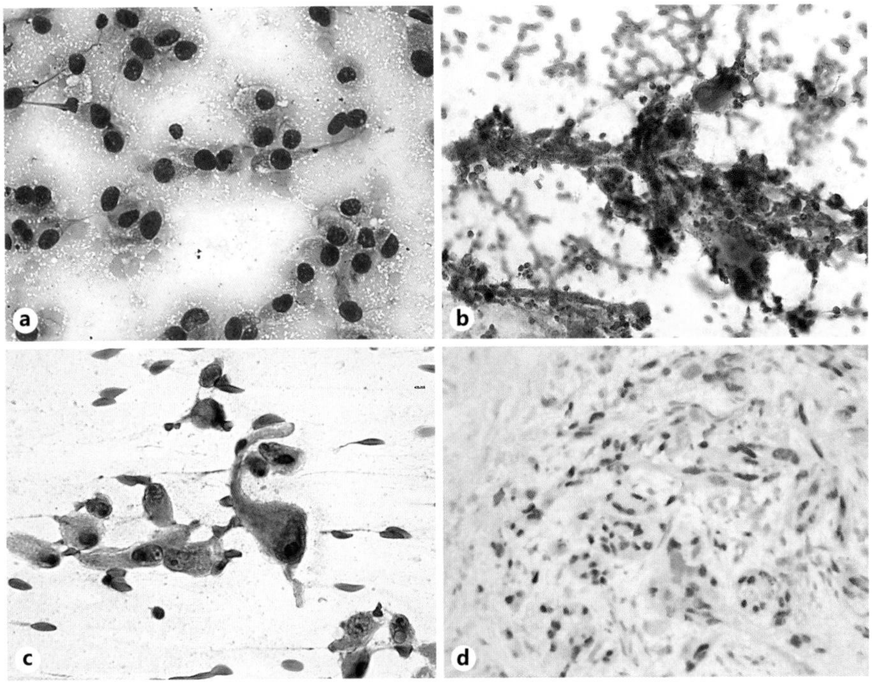

Fig. 10. Melanoma. **a** Spindled and epithelioid cells. Diff-Quik stain. **b** Abundant melanin pigment. Papanicolaou stain. **c** Malignant cells with cytoplasmic processes. Pleomorphic nuclei with prominent nuclei. One cell has an intranuclear inclusion. Papanicolaou stain. **d** SOX10 shows strong nuclear expression. Cell block, immunoperoxidase stain.

Key Pathological Findings
- Depend on the primary site
- Ovarian serous carcinomas are pleomorphic with papillary aggregates, or sheets of malignant cells

Ancillary Studies
Gynecological primaries express PAX8 (Fig. 9c). In addition, ovarian serous primaries are also positive for p53 (Fig. 9d) and WT1 (Fig. 9e).

Differential Diagnosis
PDAC is negative for PAX8 and WT1.

Skin Primaries: Melanoma
Melanoma is the most frequent skin cancer to metastasize to the pancreas. Aspirates of melanoma are cellular and dyshesive. The cells are overtly malignant in appearance, with nuclear pleomorphism, and prominent nucleoli (Fig. 10a–c). There is typically an admixture of epithelioid and spindle-shaped cells. The presence of melanin pigment is diagnostic.

Key Pathological Findings
- Dyshesive cell population or small clusters
- Nuclei eccentric or centrally placed
- Pleomorphic nuclei with prominent nucleoli or intranuclear inclusions

Ancillary Studies
Immunohistochemistry for melanoma markers including SOX10 (Fig. 10d), S100, HMB45, MelanA/MART1, and melanocyte inducing transcription factor (MITF) can be used to confirm the diagnosis of melanoma.

Differential Diagnosis
Melanoma has been described as the great mimicker. However, it is unlikely to be mistaken for PDAC, not otherwise specified. The differential diagnosis could include an undifferentiated, sarcomatoid-appearing carcinoma. Immunohistochemistry for melanoma markers will confirm the diagnosis.

Merkel Cell Carcinoma
Merkel cell carcinoma has been reported as a metastasis to the pancreas (Fig. 11a). The morphology overlaps with small-cell carcinomas from other body sites, and with primary pancreatic small-cell carcinoma.

Key Pathological Findings
- Dyshesive cell population
- Small cells with scant cytoplasm

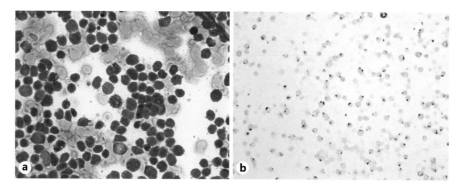

Fig. 11. Merkel cell carcinoma. **a** The malignant cells are small, with scant to absent cytoplasm, and angulated nuclei with molding. A mitosis is identified in the center. The morphology is similar to small-cell neuroendocrine carcinoma. Diff-Quik stain. **b** CK20 is expressed in a dot-like perinuclear pattern. Cell block, immunoperoxidase.

- High N:C ratio
- Nuclear molding
- Hyperchromatic nuclei

Ancillary Studies
Merkel cell carcinomas express CK20 in a dot-like, paranuclear pattern (Fig. 11b), and are positive for the Merkel cell polyoma virus, and negative for CK7 and TTF1 [37].

Differential Diagnosis
The key differential diagnosis for Merkel cell carcinoma is small-cell neuroendocrine carcinoma. Ancillary testing will differentiate between the two, as Merkel cell carcinoma has a unique phenotype as described above.

Less Common Carcinomas
Carcinomas with a hepatoid morphology present a unique challenge, as there are reported cases of hepatoid pancreatic adenocarcinoma [38], which overlap in morphological and immunophenotypical features with primary hepatocellular carcinoma. Pancreatic hepatoid carcinomas often have other components, such as typical adenocarcinoma, neuroendocrine, or acinar components [38], and these features can assist with identifying a primary. Given the rarity of hepatoid pancreatic carcinoma, a carcinoma in the pancreas with hepatoid features is a metastasis until proven otherwise. In situ hybridization for albumin mRNA has been reported to be specific for carcinomas originating in the liver, and could be useful to exclude hepatoid PDAC or confirm primary cholangiocarcinoma [39, 40].

Rare and Non-Epithelial Malignancies
The literature is replete with case reports of rare malignancies metastasizing to the pancreas. Utilization of an antibody panel that includes site-specific markers is essential to the work-up. Other site-specific markers are NKX3.1 for prostate, and PAX8, TTF1, and thyroglobulin for thyroid carcinoma [41]. Sarcomas are not uncommon, and the morphological differential diagnosis includes undifferentiated carcinoma of the pancreas. Undifferentiated carcinomas of the pancreas coexpress cytokeratins and vimentin, whereas most sarcomas are negative for cytokeratins. The FNA case series included some unusual metastases which are presented in Table 2. The reader should always consider rare malignancies metastasizing to the pancreas when encountering malignancies with an unusual morphology in the pancreas.

Hematopoietic Malignancies

Overview
All hematopoietic malignancies, including non-Hodgkin's and Hodgkin's lymphomas, leukemias, and plasmacytomas, have been reported secondarily involving the pancreas [1]. The prevalent mode of involvement is extension from retroperitoneal lymph nodes, the duodenum, or adjacent peripancreatic lymph nodes [42]. Non-Hodgkin's lymphoma is the most common, and one-third of patients with non-Hodgkin's lymphoma reportedly have pancreatic involvement.

Primary pancreatic lymphoma is extremely rare. It can be diagnosed only if the following criteria are met: (1) absence of superficial lymphadenopathy or mediastinal adenopathy, (2) normal leukocyte count in the peripheral blood, (3) main mass located in the pancreas with lymph nodal involvement confined to peripancreatic lymph nodes, and (4) no hepatic or splenic involvement [42]. Most primary pancreatic lymphomas are large B-cell lymphomas. Both primary pancreatic lymphoma and secondary pancreatic involvement may present as a solitary mass, for which

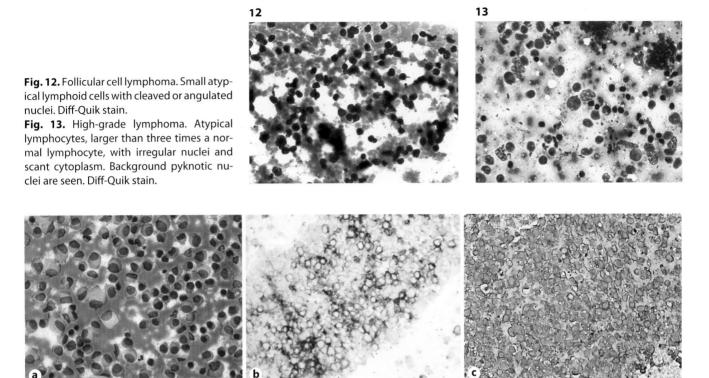

Fig. 12. Follicular cell lymphoma. Small atypical lymphoid cells with cleaved or angulated nuclei. Diff-Quik stain.

Fig. 13. High-grade lymphoma. Atypical lymphocytes, larger than three times a normal lymphocyte, with irregular nuclei and scant cytoplasm. Background pyknotic nuclei are seen. Diff-Quik stain.

Fig. 14. Plasmacytoma. **a** Single cells with eccentric nuclei. Diff-Quik stain. **b** Cytoplasmic expression for CD138. Cell block, immunoperoxidase stain. **c** Immunohistochemistry for kappa shows strong cytoplasmic expression, confirming kappa light chain restriction. Cell block, immunoperoxidase.

the imaging differential diagnosis is a primary pancreatic neoplasm. Primary pancreatic lymphomas are less likely to have vascular invasion than PDAC, and less likely to present with obstruction of the MPD [43].

Cytology smears are typically cellular and composed of a dyshesive, monotonous cell pattern. Lymphoglandular bodies may be present on the slide background. The size and cytological features of the malignant lymphocytes is predicated by the type of lymphoma. The cytoplasm is scant to visibly absent. The nuclei may be round, as in small lymphocytic lymphoma (Fig. 12), or angulated. The lymphocytes in large-cell lymphoma are 3–4 times the size of normal lymphocytes, and they have single or multiple nucleoli, and nuclear membrane irregularities (Fig. 13). Necrosis and karyorrhexis are features of high-grade lymphomas.

Key Pathological Findings
- Dyshesive cells
- Lymphoglandular bodies
- Cell size and nuclear features depend on the specific subtypes

Ancillary Studies

Diagnosis of hematopoietic diseases depends on immunophenotyping, either by flow cytometry or immunohistochemistry, and cytogenetics. On-site evaluations showing a lymphoid population suspicious for lymphoma should prompt additional sample collection for flow cytometry. Ancillary studies for lymphoma work-up can be successfully performed from EUS-FNA samples [44]. Diagnosis of lymphoma involving the pancreas and primary pancreatic lymphoma can be highly accurate when coupled with flow cytometry and cytogenetics [45, 46]. The classification of lymphomas is described in detail in the 2016 revision of the WHO classification of lymphomas [47], and is beyond the scope of this chapter.

Differential Diagnosis

The differential diagnosis is primarily with solid, cellular neoplasms of the pancreas, which all produce cellular, dyshesive monotonous smears. Acinar cell carcinoma, solid pseudopapillary neoplasm, and PanNETs will have cell groups with cellular cohesion, and more abundant cytoplasm in contrast to lymphoma. Each of these has distinguishing cytoplasmic and nuclear features. When in doubt, immunohistochemical panels, as described in the chapter on non-ductal neoplasms by Dhillon [this vol., pp. 92–108], will be useful to differentiate these neoplasms from lymphomas.

Plasmacytomas rarely involve the pancreas, and a few reports have described the clinical and cytopathological findings (Fig. 14a) [48–50]. They have also been identified in a case series of metastatic disease [13, 16, 20]. Plasmacytomas may present with biliary tract obstruction. The key differential diagnosis is with PanNET [49], which is plasmacytoid in appearance. Plasmacytomas are positive for CD138 (Fig. 14b) and show light chain restriction with kappa (Fig. 14c) or lambda. They are negative for cytokeratins and neuroendocrine markers. PanNET in the pancreas is more common than plasmacytoma, and therefore should be considered first.

Disclosure Statement

The author has no conflicts of interest to disclose.

References

1 Hruban RH, Pitman MB, Klimstra DS: In: Albores-Saavedra J, Owen DA (eds): Tumors of the Pancreas. AFIP Atlas of Tumor Pathology. Washington, American Registry of Pathology, 2007, pp 325–333.

2 Raymond SLT, Yugawa D, Chang KHF, Ena B, Tauchi-Nishi PS: Metastatic neoplasms to the pancreas diagnosed by fine-needle aspiration/biopsy cytology: a 15-year retrospective analysis. Diagn Cytopathol 2017;45:771–783.

3 Tan CH, Tamm EP, Marcal L, Balachandran A, Charnsangavej C, Vikram R, Bhosale P: Imaging features of hematogenous metastases to the pancreas: pictorial essay. Cancer Imaging 2011;11:9–15.

4 Ahmed S, Johnson PT, Hruban R, Fishman EK: Metastatic disease to the pancreas: pathologic spectrum and CT patterns. Abdom Imaging 2013;38:144–153.

5 Krishna SG, Bhattacharya A, Ross WA, Ladha H, Porter K, Bhutani MS, Lee JH: Pretest prediction and diagnosis of metastatic lesions to the pancreas by endoscopic ultrasound-guided fine needle aspiration. J Gastroenterol Hepatol 2015;30:1552–1560.

6 Eloubeidi MA, Tamhane AR, Buxbaum JL: Unusual, metastatic, or neuroendocrine tumor of the pancreas: a diagnosis with endoscopic ultrasound-guided fine-needle aspiration and immunohistochemistry. Saudi J Gastroenterol 2012;18:99–105.

7 Hijioka S, Matsuo K, Mizuno N, Hara K, Mekky MA, Vikram B, Hosoda W, Yatabe Y, Shimizu Y, Kondo S, Tajika M, Niwa Y, Tamada K, Yamao K: Role of endoscopic ultrasound and endoscopic ultrasound-guided fine-needle aspiration in diagnosing metastasis to the pancreas: a tertiary center experience. Pancreatology 2011;11:390–398.

8 Gagovic V, Spier BJ, DeLee RJ, Barancin C, Lindstrom M, Einstein M, Byrne S, Harter J, Agni R, Pfau PR, Frick TJ, Soni A, Gopal DV: Endoscopic ultrasound fine-needle aspiration characteristics of primary adenocarcinoma versus other malignant neoplasms of the pancreas. Can J Gastroenterol 2012;26:691–696.

9 Edgren M, Westlin JE, Kalkner KM, Sundin A, Nilsson S: [¹¹¹In-DPTA-D-Phe¹]-octreotide scintigraphy in the management of patients with advanced renal cell carcinoma. Cancer Biother Radiopharm 1999;14:59–64.

10 Benning TL, Silverman JF, Berns LA, Geisinger KR: Fine needle aspiration of metastatic and hematologic malignancies clinically mimicking pancreatic carcinoma. Acta Cytol 1992;36:471–476.

11 Carson HJ, Green LK, Castelli MJ, Reyes CV, Prinz RA, Gattuso P: Utilization of fine-needle aspiration biopsy in the diagnosis of metastatic tumors to the pancreas. Diagn Cytopathol 1995;12:8–13.

12 Fritscher-Ravens A, Sriram PV, Krause C, Atay Z, Jaeckle S, Thonke F, Brand B, Bohnacker S, Soehendra N: Detection of pancreatic metastases by EUS-guided fine-needle aspiration. Gastrointest Endosc 2001;53:65–70.

13 Alomari AK, Ustun B, Aslanian HR, Ge X, Chhieng D, Cai G: Endoscopic ultrasound-guided fine-needle aspiration diagnosis of secondary tumors involving the pancreas: an institution's experience. Cytojournal 2016;13:1.

14 Ardengh JC, Lopes CV, Kemp R, Venco F, de Lima-Filho ER, dos Santos JS: Accuracy of endoscopic ultrasound-guided fine-needle aspiration in the suspicion of pancreatic metastases. BMC Gastroenterol 2013;13:63.

15 Atiq M, Bhutani MS, Ross WA, Raju GS, Gong Y, Tamm EP, Javle M, Wang X, Lee JH: Role of endoscopic ultrasonography in evaluation of metastatic lesions to the pancreas: a tertiary cancer center experience. Pancreas 2013;42:516–523.

16 Betes M, Gonzalez Vazquez S, Bojorquez A, Lozano MD, Echeveste JI, Garcia Albarran L, Munoz Navas M, Subtil JC: Metastatic tumors in the pancreas: the role of endoscopic ultrasound-guided fine-needle aspiration. Rev Esp Enferm Dig 2019;111:345–350.

17 De Witt J, Jowell P, Leblanc J, McHenry L, McGreevy K, Cramer H, Volmar K, Sherman S, Gress F: EUS-guided FNA of pancreatic metastases: a multicenter experience. Gastrointest Endosc 2005;61:689–696.

18 El Hajj II, LeBlanc JK, Sherman S, Al-Haddad MA, Cote GA, McHenry L, DeWitt JM: Endoscopic ultrasound-guided biopsy of pancreatic metastases: a large single-center experience. Pancreas 2013;42:524–530.

19 Gilbert CM, Monaco SE, Cooper ST, Khalbuss WE: Endoscopic ultrasound-guided fine-needle aspiration of metastases to the pancreas: a study of 25 cases. Cytojournal 2011;8:7.

20 Layfield LJ, Hirschowitz SL, Adler DG: Metastatic disease to the pancreas documented by endoscopic ultrasound guided fine-needle aspiration: a seven-year experience. Diagn Cytopathol 2012;40:228–233.

21 Mesa H, Stelow EB, Stanley MW, Mallery S, Lai R, Bardales RH: Diagnosis of nonprimary pancreatic neoplasms by endoscopic ultrasound-guided fine-needle aspiration. Diagn Cytopathol 2004;31:313–318.

22 Olson MT, Wakely PE Jr, Ali SZ: Metastases to the pancreas diagnosed by fine-needle aspiration. Acta Cytol 2013;57:473–480.

23 Sekulic M, Amin K, Mettler T, Miller LK, Mallery S, Stewart JR: Pancreatic involvement by metastasizing neoplasms as determined by endoscopic ultrasound-guided fine needle aspiration: a clinicopathologic characterization. Diagn Cytopathol 2017;45:418–425.

24 Smith AL, Odronic SI, Springer BS, Reynolds JP: Solid tumor metastases to the pancreas diagnosed by FNA: a single-institution experience and review of the literature. Cancer Cytopathol 2015;123:347–355.

25 Volmar KE, Jones CK, Xie HB: Metastases in the pancreas from nonhematologic neoplasms: report of 20 cases evaluated by fine-needle aspiration. Diagn Cytopathol 2004;31:216–220.

26 Waters L, Si Q, Caraway N, Mody D, Staerkel G, Sneige N: Secondary tumors of the pancreas diagnosed by endoscopic ultrasound-guided fine-needle aspiration: a 10-year experience. Diagn Cytopathol 2014;42:738–743.

27 Hou Y, Shen R, Tonkovich D, Li Z: Endoscopic ultrasound-guided fine-needle aspiration diagnosis of secondary tumors involving pancreas: an institution's experience. J Am Soc Cytopathol 2018;7:261–267.

28 Ballarin R, Spaggiari M, Cautero N, De Ruvo N, Montalti R, Longo C, Pecchi A, Giacobazzi P, De Marco G, D'Amico G, Gerunda GE, Di Benedetto F: Pancreatic metastases from renal cell carcinoma: the state of the art. World J Gastroenterol 2011;17:4747–4756.

29 Centeno BA, Stelow EB, Pitman MB: Pancreatic Cytohistology. Cytohistology of Small Tissue Samples. Cambridge, Cambridge University Press, 2015, pp 154–163.

30 Lew M, Foo WC, Roh MH: Diagnosis of metastatic renal cell carcinoma on fine-needle aspiration cytology. Arch Pathol Lab Med 2014;138:1278–1285.

31 Bishop JA, Sharma R, Illei PB: Napsin A and thyroid transcription factor-1 expression in carcinomas of the lung, breast, pancreas, colon, kidney, thyroid, and malignant mesothelioma. Hum Pathol 2010;41:20–25.

32 Matoso A, Singh K, Jacob R, Greaves WO, Tavares R, Noble L, Resnick MB, Delellis RA, Wang LJ: Comparison of thyroid transcription factor-1 expression by 2 monoclonal antibodies in pulmonary and nonpulmonary primary tumors. Appl Immunohistochem Mol Morphol 2010;18:142–149.

33 Kaufmann O, Dietel M: Expression of thyroid transcription factor-1 in pulmonary and extrapulmonary small cell carcinomas and other neuroendocrine carcinomas of various primary sites. Histopathology 2000;36:415–420.

34 Chen ZE, Lin F: Application of immunohistochemistry in gastrointestinal and liver neoplasms: new markers and evolving practice. Arch Pathol Lab Med 2015;139:14–23.

35 Adsay NV, Merati K, Basturk O, Iacobuzio-Donahue C, Levi E, Cheng JD, Sarkar FH, Hruban RH, Klimstra DS: Pathologically and biologically distinct types of epithelium in intraductal papillary mucinous neoplasms: delineation of an "intestinal" pathway of carcinogenesis in the pancreas. Am J Surg Pathol 2004;28:839–848.

36 Miettinen M, McCue PA, Sarlomo-Rikala M, Rys J, Czapiewski P, Wazny K, Langfort R, Waloszczyk P, Biernat W, Lasota J, Wang Z: GATA3: a multispecific but potentially useful marker in surgical pathology: a systematic analysis of 2,500 epithelial and nonepithelial tumors. Am J Surg Pathol 2014; 38:13–22.

37 Li L, Molberg K, Cheedella N, Thibodeaux J, Hinson S, Lucas E: The diagnostic utility of Merkel cell polyomavirus immunohistochemistry in a fine needle aspirate of metastatic Merkel cell carcinoma of unknown primary to the pancreas. Diagn Cytopathol 2018;46:67–71.

38 Marchegiani G, Gareer H, Parisi A, Capelli P, Bassi C, Salvia R: Pancreatic hepatoid carcinoma: a review of the literature. Dig Surg 2013;30:425–433.

39 Ferrone CR, Ting DT, Shahid M, Konstantinidis IT, Sabbatino F, Goyal L, Rice-Stitt T, Mubeen A, Arora K, Bardeesey N, Miura J, Gamblin TC, Zhu AX, Borger D, Lillemoe KD, Rivera MN, Deshpande V: The ability to diagnose intrahepatic cholangiocarcinoma definitively using novel branched DNA-enhanced albumin RNA in situ hybridization technology. Ann Surg Oncol 2016; 23:290–296.

40 Shahid M, Mubeen A, Tse J, Kakar S, Bateman AC, Borger D, Rivera MN, Ting DT, Deshpande V: Branched chain in situ hybridization for albumin as a marker of hepatocellular differentiation: evaluation of manual and automated in situ hybridization platforms. Am J Surg Pathol 2015;39:25–34.

41 Cowan ML, VandenBussche CJ: Cancer of unknown primary: ancillary testing of cytologic and small biopsy specimens in the era of targeted therapy. Cancer Cytopathol 2018;126(suppl 8):724–737.

42 Saif MW: Primary pancreatic lymphomas. JOP 2006;7:262–273.

43 Johnson EA, Benson ME, Guda N, Pfau PR, Frick TJ, Gopal DV: Differentiating primary pancreatic lymphoma from adenocarcinoma using endoscopic ultrasound characteristics and flow cytometry: a case-control study. Endosc Ultrasound 2014;3:221–225.

44 Jin M, Wakely PE Jr: Endoscopic/endobronchial ultrasound-guided fine needle aspiration and ancillary techniques, particularly flow cytometry, in diagnosing deep-seated lymphomas. Acta Cytol 2016;60:326–335.

45 Sadaf S, Loya A, Akhtar N, Yusuf MA: Role of endoscopic ultrasound-guided-fine needle aspiration biopsy in the diagnosis of lymphoma of the pancreas: a clinicopathological study of nine cases. Cytopathology 2017;28:536–541.

46 Nayer H, Weir EG, Sheth S, Ali SZ: Primary pancreatic lymphomas: a cytopathologic analysis of a rare malignancy. Cancer 2004;102:315–321.

47 Swerdlow SH, Campo E, Pileri SA, Harris NL, Stein H, Siebert R, Advani R, Ghielmini M, Salles GA, Zelenetz AD, Jaffe ES: The 2016 revision of the World Health Organization classification of lymphoid neoplasms. Blood 2016;127:2375–2390.

48 Roh YH, Hwang SY, Lee SM, Im JW, Kim JS, Kwon KA, Song JY, Jeong SY: Extramedullary plasmacytoma of the pancreas diagnosed using endoscopic ultrasonography-guided fine needle aspiration. Clin Endosc 2014;47:115–118.

49 Dodd LG, Evans DB, Symmans F, Katz RL: Fine-needle aspiration of pancreatic extramedullary plasmacytoma: possible confusion with islet cell tumor. Diagn Cytopathol 1994;10:371–375.

50 Lopes da Silva R: Pancreatic involvement by plasma cell neoplasms. J Gastrointest Cancer 2012;43:157–167.

Prof. Barbara A. Centeno
Moffitt Cancer Center
12902 USF Magnolia Drive
Tampa, FL 33612 (USA)
barbara.centeno@moffitt.org

Published online: September 29, 2020

Centeno BA, Dhillon J (eds): Pancreatic Tumors. Monogr Clin Cytol. Basel, Karger, 2020, vol 26, pp 122–128
(DOI:10.1159/000455739)

Mesenchymal Tumors of the Pancreas

Jasreman Dhillon[a, b]

[a]Department of Anatomic Pathology, Moffitt Cancer Center, Tampa, FL, USA; [b]Department of Oncologic Sciences and Pathology,
University of South Florida, Tampa, FL, USA

Abstract

This chapter describes the mesenchymal tumors of the pancreas which are of rare occurrence. Mesenchymal tumors of the pancreas may be benign, of intermediate biological potential or malignant. The more commonly occurring mesenchymal tumors of the pancreas are described in this chapter along with their appropriate immunohistochemical workup and differential diagnoses.   © 2020 S. Karger AG, Basel

Primary mesenchymal tumors of the pancreas are rare with a reported incidence of 0.1% of pancreatic sarcoma diagnosed after autopsy [1]. Benign mesenchymal tumors comprise lymphangiomas, hemangiomas, schwannomas, solitary fibrous tumors (SFTs), adenomatoid tumor, leiomyomas, and hamartomas. Inflammatory myofibroblastic tumors (IMTs) are pseudotumors that are considered to be of intermediate biological potential due to local recurrences and rarely distant metastases. Malignant mesenchymal tumors include leiomyosarcomas, malignant peripheral nerve sheath tumors, liposarcoma, Ewing's sarcoma, and primitive neuroectodermal tumor. It is important to recognize these tumors as pancreatic primaries and distinguish them from sarcomatoid carcinomas and retroperitoneal sarcomas that secondarily involve the pancreas. Some of the more common mesenchymal tumors occurring in the pancreas are described here.

Fibroblastic and Myofibroblastic Tumors

Inflammatory Myofibroblastic Tumor

IMT, also known as inflammatory pseudotumor, is a generic term applied to a heterogeneous group of lesions occurring in various organs, which are histologically characterized by fibroblastic and myofibroblastic proliferation with inflammatory cell infiltrate [2]. IMT was originally described in the lungs and has since then been described in other organs, such as the bladder, liver, spleen, lymph nodes, gastrointestinal tract, and rarely in the pancreas. IMTs are considered by the WHO as tumors of intermediate biological potential due to local recurrences and rarely distant metastases [3].

Histology

Few cases of pancreatic IMT have been reported in the literature [4–7]. The tumors are reported to occur from 6 months up to 64 years of age. It can involve the head, body/tail, or uncinate process of the pancreas. Patients are either asymptomatic or present with abdominal pain, jaundice, or weight loss. Clinically and radiographically, IMTs may resemble pancreatic adenocarcinoma.

The tumor is composed of myofibroblastic spindle cells which may have a storiform pattern. Admixed is inflammatory infiltrate composed of plasma cells, lymphocytes, eosinophils, and histiocytes in a collagenous or myxoid background [8]. IMTs stain positive for vimentin, ALK, smooth muscle actin (SMA), and desmin. IMTs must be differentiated from chronic pancreatitis, fibrosarcoma, pancreatic carcinoma, and lymphoma [9]. IMTs are primarily treated with surgery.

Cytology

It is difficult to diagnose IMTs on cytology. Cytological smears may show the presence of bland or mildly pleomorphic spindle cells admixed with inflammatory cells composed of plasma cells, lymphocytes, eosinophils, and histiocytes. These cytological features have to be distinguished from inflammatory lesions such as autoimmune pancreatitis and chronic pancreatitis. A suggestion of IMT can be made on cytological smears with a comment that other differential diagnoses cannot be entirely excluded. The entire lesion has to be histologically examined utilizing appropriate immunostains to confirm the diagnosis of IMT and rule out other differential diagnoses.

Key Cytological Features
- Mildly pleomorphic spindle cells admixed with inflammatory cells
- Elongated cytoplasmic tails
- Large polygonal cells
- Spindle cells are positive for ALK, SMA, desmin
- Correlation with clinical and radiographic findings is necessary to exclude other diagnostic entities

Solitary Fibrous Tumor

SFTs are mesenchymal tumors presumed to be of fibroblastic differentiation. SFTs most commonly affect adults and can occur at any site [10]. Pancreatic SFTs are rare; less than 20 cases have been reported in the literature. The tumors are predominantly seen in adult women and may present as incidental findings or with abdominal pain.

Histology

The tumors are located in the head or body of the pancreas and range in size from 1.5 up to 18.5 cm [11]. The tumors are well-circumscribed, partially encapsulated masses. The cut surface can be multinodular, white, and firm. Histologically, SFT is composed of bland spindle cells, with elongated nuclei, which exhibit a storiform pattern with alternating hypocellular and hypercellular areas (Fig. 1a). Intermixed are thick bands of collagen and numerous branching hemangiopericytomatous blood vessels. Mitotic figures are rare. Other spindle cell tumors, such as leiomyoma, leiomyosarcoma, fibrosarcoma, and gastrointestinal stromal tumor (GIST), are in the differential diagnosis. Immunohistochemical stains are key in diagnosing SFTs as these tumors are positive for CD34, Bcl2, and STAT6, and are generally negative for cytokeratins, smooth muscle markers, CD117, and S100.

Cytology

The smears are composed of clusters of bland spindle cells with little cytologic atypia. Single cells are present in the background (Fig. 1b, c). Dense, ropy collagen is present in between the spindle cells. No necrosis is present in the background [12]. Immunostains as described above are key to the diagnosis.

Key Cytological Features
- Clusters as well as single cells composed of bland spindle cells with fusiform nucleus
- Dense, ropy collagen
- Naked nuclei
- SFTs are positive for CD34, Bcl2, and STAT6

Schwannoma

Overview

Schwannomas are peripheral nerve sheath tumors that arise from the Schwann cells [13]. Schwannomas occur sporadically or can be associated with neurofibromatosis type II. Pancreatic schwannomas are very rare tumors, with 65 cases reported in the English literature over the past 40 years [14]. The patients range in age from 20 years up to 87 years. Patients may either be asymptomatic or present with abdominal pain, weight loss, back pain, and/or nausea/vomiting. The majority of the tumors are located in the head followed by the body of the pancreas. Most of the cases are benign, with only 4 malignant schwannomas of the pancreas reported [15–19]. Surgery is the optimal treatment and patients generally have a good prognosis following complete tumor resection. The recurrence rate is extremely low [20, 21].

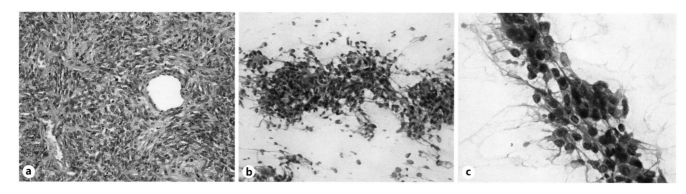

Fig. 1. SFT. **a** Bland-appearing spindle cells exhibiting a storiform pattern. HE stain, ×20. **b** Cluster of tumor cells composed of spindle cells and few scattered single cells in the background. HE stain, ×20. **c** Tumor cells with mildly pleomorphic, oval nuclei with inconspicuous nucleoli. HE stain, ×40. Images courtesy of Dr. Marilyn Bui.

Histology

Tumors range in size from 1 up to 20 cm and can present as either solid or cystic masses [14]. The tumors are surrounded by a thin capsule and are composed of spindle cells with palisading and fascicular arrangement. The tumor typically shows hypercellular (Antoni A) and hypocellular (Antoni B) areas. The hypercellular foci may show peripheral palisading of the tumor nuclei and Verocay bodies. Myxoid stroma is present in the hypocellular foci. The tumor may undergo cystic degeneration, hemorrhage, and calcifications. The majority of the pancreatic schwannomas are benign. Malignant schwannomas are characterized by nuclear enlargement and hyperchromasia, increased mitotic activity, and pleomorphic spindle cells infiltrating into the surrounding organs. Immunohistochemical stains show the tumor cells to be strongly positive for S100 and SOX10, and negative for actin, smooth muscle myosin, desmin, CD34, and CD117.

Cytology

The smears are moderately cellular and are composed of bland spindle cells. The neoplastic cells form large, cohesive tissue fragments [22]. The tissue fragments exhibit nuclear palisading and a wavy fibrillary cytoplasm (Fig. 2a, b). Since most of the schwannomas are benign, mitotic figures and necrosis are generally absent. Immunohistochemical stains, as described above, are needed to make a diagnosis of schwannoma.

Key Cytological Features
- Fragments of large cohesive bland spindle cells
- Wavy nuclei
- Wavy, fibrillary cytoplasm
- Nuclear palisading
- Tumor cells are strongly positive for S100 and SOX10

Leiomyoma and Leiomyosarcoma

Overview

Pancreatic leiomyomas are extremely rare [23, 24]. Of the 3 cases reported in the literature, all of these were in the head of the pancreas [23–25]. Two of the patients were female (62 and 72 years of age) and 1 was a 52-year-old male.

Pancreatic leiomyosarcomas are relatively more common, with close to 70 cases reported in the literature [26]. Pancreatic leiomyosarcoma is the most common pancreatic sarcoma [1, 27]. It has an equal sex distribution with a median age of presentation at 55 years. The tumors are equally distributed between the head and the body-tail of the pancreas. Presenting symptoms range from asymptomatic for the smaller, incidentally discovered tumors, to abdominal pain, abdominal mass, weight loss, and jaundice. Tumor sizes have been reported to range from 1 up to 30 cm. Surgery with free tumor margins is the standard treatment for leiomyosarcomas localized to the pancreas.

Histology

Leiomyomas are spindle cell neoplasms that are composed of bland tumor cells without necrosis, mitotic figures, and hemorrhagic foci. Immunohistochemical stains are very helpful in making a diagnosis of leiomyoma and are positive for SMA, muscle-specific actin (HHF35), and desmin, and are negative for CD117, DOG1, CD34, and S100. Leiomyomas are benign tumors generally with a good prognosis. Of

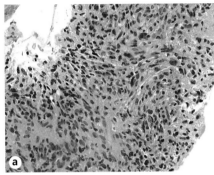
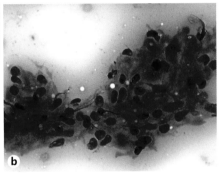

Fig. 2. Schwannoma. **a** A large cluster of tumor cells with spindled nuclei. Diff-Quik stain, ×20. **b** A cluster of spindle cells with oval to round nuclei and abundant fibrillary cytoplasm. Diff-Quik stain, ×40.

Fig. 3. Leiomyosarcoma. **a** Spindle cell neoplasm with oval to irregular moderately pleomorphic nuclei. HE stain, ×20. **b** A cluster of spindle cells with blunt-ended oval nuclei and a moderate amount of cytoplasm. Diff-Quik stain, ×40. Images courtesy of Dr. Marilyn Bui.

the 3 patients, 1 was placed on active observation without any surgical intervention, and 2 had surgery, Whipple's procedure, and enucleation of the tumor.

Leiomyosarcomas are spindle cell tumors with pleomorphism, necrosis, and mitoses including atypical mitotic figures (Fig. 3a). Muscle markers are positive as described above.

Cytology

The smears show a spindle cell neoplasm. In leiomyomas the spindle cells are bland with cigar-shaped nuclei and a moderate amount of cytoplasm. Mitotic figures and necrosis are absent. Leiomyosarcomas show sheets of interlacing pleomorphic spindle cells with indistinct cytoplasmic borders (Fig. 3b). Bare, pleomorphic nuclei with blunted ends may be present in the background [28, 29]. Mitotic figures are present.

Key Cytological Features
- Leiomyomas show fragments of bland spindle cells without necrosis and mitosis
- Leiomyosarcomas show pleomorphic spindle cells including cells with naked nuclei and mitotic figures
- Cigar-shaped nuclei
- Tumor cells are positive for SMA, HHF35, and desmin

Tumors of Perivascular Epithelioid Cells

Overview
Tumors of the perivascular epithelioid cells (PEComas) represent a family of neoplasms that are characterized by immunohistochemical evidence of dual myomelanocytic differentiation [30]. Angiomyolipoma, clear cell "sugar" tumor, and lymphangioleiomyomatosis are lesions that are commonly included in this family. Histologically comparable lesions arise from intraabdominal and somatic soft tissues, the uterus, urinary bladder, gastrointestinal tract, and pancreas.

Less than 20 cases of pancreatic PEComas (perivascular epithelioid cell tumors) have been described in the literature. None of them have been reported to be associated with tuberous sclerosis. Most cases arise in adult females and are located in the head, body, or uncinate process of the pancreas. Patients commonly present with either abdominal pain or are asymptomatic. Two cases have been reported to have metastasized to the liver.

Histology
Pancreatic PEComas vary in size from 1.5 up to 10 cm. The cut surface is tan white and soft. Larger tumors may undergo cystic changes secondary to necrosis and hemorrhage [31]. Histologically, the tumor cells are either nested or pres-

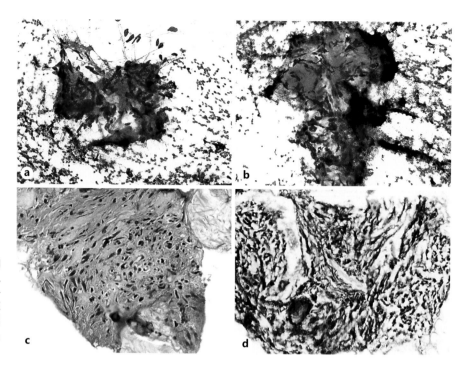

Fig. 4. GIST. **a**, **b** Cluster of spindle cells and background stroma. Diff-Quik stain, ×20. **c** Cell block section with spindle cells embedded in a background of myxoid stroma. HE stain, ×40. **d** DOG1 immunohistochemical stain diffusely positive in the tumor cells, ×40.

ent in diffuse sheets. The tumor cells may be spindled, epithelioid, or a mixture of the two and contain a granular eosinophilic to clear cytoplasm. The tumor cells can be seen concentrically present around few blood vessels. Malignant cases frequently show a marked pleomorphism, readily identified mitoses, and necrosis. The tumor cells express melanocytic markers, such as HMB45, melan-A, and MITF, and smooth muscle markers such as SMA.

Cytology

Smears show fragments of spindle cells with abundant clear to eosinophilic cytoplasm with indistinct cytoplasmic borders [32]. Epithelioid tumor cells may be admixed. Single cells are present in the background. Nuclei are oval and may vary in size. The tumor has to be distinguished from other pancreatic tumors such as neuroendocrine tumor, solid pseudopapillary tumor, and GIST. PEComas are negative for epithelial and neuroendocrine markers and are usually negative for CD117 and do not exhibit the c-kit mutation.

Key Cytological Features
• Fragments of spindle to epithelioid cells
• Moderate to abundant granular, clear to eosinophilic cytoplasm
• Coexpress melanocytic and smooth muscle markers

Gastrointestinal Stromal Tumors

Overview
GIST is a mesenchymal tumor that predominantly involves the stomach and small intestine. Less than 5% of cases are extragastrointestinal, with pancreatic tumors being extremely rare [33]. GISTs occur primarily in older patients of either sex. They are characterized by the expression of CD117, a protein encoded by the c-kit gene.

Histology
Pancreatic GISTs can be solid, cystic, or both. Some of the larger tumors may grow up to 30 cm in size and exhibit secondary degenerative changes such as foci of central necrosis, hemorrhage, and cystic change. The tumors can involve the head, body, or tail of the pancreas.

Pancreatic GISTs are predominantly composed of spindle cells that are arranged in short fascicles and whorls. The cytoplasm is somewhat paler than smooth muscle tumors and is fibrillary in appearance.

Some of the tumors may have atypia and mitotic figures. Foci of necrosis may be admixed. GISTs of epithelioid type are composed of rounded cells with an eosinophilic or clear cytoplasm. Some of the tumors may have both spindled as well as epithelioid cells [34]. Nuclei are oval to round in shape and may exhibit palisading. Prominent myxoid stroma is occasionally present in these tumors. Pancreatic GISTs most commonly metastasize to the liver.

In general, the c-kit gene is expressed in 95% of GISTs; 60–70% of GISTs are CD34 positive and have low expression of SMA (30–40%), desmin (<5%), NSE, and S100 (<5%) [35]. DOG1 and CD117 stain >95% of GISTs between them.

Pancreatic GISTs are primarily treated by surgery. Advanced, unresectable GISTs have been treated with the tyrosine kinase inhibitor imatinib [35].

Cytology

EUS-FNA is an efficient diagnostic tool for preoperative diagnosis of pancreatic GISTs. There are a handful of case reports in the literature describing cytological features of pancreatic GISTs [33, 36]. The tumors are described as being composed of spindle-shaped cells arranged in small clusters and sheets (Fig. 4a, b). One of the cases had a myxoid background [37]. Immunohistochemical stains are required to make this diagnosis and rule out other spindle cell tumors (Fig. 4c, d).

Key Cytological Features

- Spindle cells present in small clusters which may exhibit palisading
- Background may be myxoid
- Tumor cells are positive for CD117, DOG1

Other Mesenchymal Tumors

Other rare mesenchymal tumors include benign entities such as lymphangioma, hemangioma, adenomatoid tumor, and hamartomas, and malignant tumors such as malignant peripheral nerve sheath tumors, liposarcomas, Ewing's sarcomas, and primitive neuroectodermal tumors [38]. It is important to correctly recognize these entities for adequate patient management.

Disclosure Statement

The author has no conflicts of interest to disclose.

References

1 Baylor SM, Berg JW: Cross-classification and survival characteristics of 5,000 cases of cancer of the pancreas. J Surg Oncol 1973;5:335–358.

2 Yamamoto H, Yamaguchi H, Aishima S, Oda Y, Kohashi K, Oshiro Y, et al: Inflammatory myofibroblastic tumor versus IgG4-related sclerosing disease and inflammatory pseudotumor: a comparative clinicopathologic study. Am J Surg Pathol 2009;33:1330–1340.

3 Coffin CM, Watterson J, Priest JR, Dehner LP: Extrapulmonary inflammatory myofibroblastic tumor (inflammatory pseudotumor). A clinicopathologic and immunohistochemical study of 84 cases. Am J Surg Pathol 1995;19:859–872.

4 Pungpapong S, Geiger XJ, Raimondo M: Inflammatory myofibroblastic tumor presenting as a pancreatic mass: a case report and review of the literature. JOP 2004;5:360–367.

5 Wreesmann V, van Eijik CHJ, Naus DCWH, Velthuysen M-LF, Jeekel J, Mooi WJ: Inflammatory pseudotumour (inflammatory myofibroblastic tumour) of the pancreas: a report of six cases associated with obliterative phlebitis. Histopathology 2001;38:105–110.

6 Walsh SV, Evangelista F, Khettry U: Inflammatory myofibroblastic tumor of the pancreaticobiliary region. Am J Surg Pathol 1998;22:412–418.

7 Tomazic A, Gvardijancic D, Maucec J, Homan M: Inflammatory myofibroblastic tumor of the pancreatic head – a case report of a 6 months old child and review of the literature. Radiol Oncol 2015;49:265–270.

8 Coffin CM, Humphrey PA, Dehner LP: Extrapulmonary inflammatory myofibroblastic tumor: a clinical and pathological survey. Semin Diagn Pathol 1998;15:85–101.

9 Meis JM, Enzinger FM: Inflammatory fibrosarcoma of the mesentery and retroperitoneum. A tumor closely simulating inflammatory pseudotumor. Am J Surg Pathol 1991;15:1146–1156.

10 Guillou L, Fletcher JA, Fletcher CDM, Mandahl N: Extrapleural solitary fibrous tumor and haemangiopericytoma; in Fletcher CDM, Unni KK, Mertens F (eds): World Health Organization Classification of Tumours. Pathology and Genetics of Tumours of Soft Tissue and Bone. Lyon, IARC Press, 2002, pp 86–90.

11 Paramythiotis D, Kofina K, Bangeas P, Tsiompanou F, Karayannopoulou G, Basdanis G: Solitary fibrous tumor of the pancreas: case report and review of the literature. World J Gastrointest Surg 2016;8:461–466.

12 Srinivasan VD, Wayne JD, Rao MS, Zynger DL: Solitary fibrous tumor of the pancreas: case report with cytologic and surgical pathology correlation and review of the literature. JOP 2008;9:526–530.

13 Das Gupta TK, Brasfield RD, Strong EW, Hajdu SI: Benign solitary schwannomas (neurilemomas). Cancer 1969;24:355–366.

14 Xu SY, Sun K, Owusu-Ansah KG, Xie HY, Zhou L, Zheng SS, Wang WL: Central pancreatectomy for pancreatic schwannoma: a case report and literature review. World J Gastroenterol 2016;22:8439–8446.

15 Stojanovic MP, Radojkovic M, Jeremic LM, Zlatic AV, Stanojevic GZ, Jovanovic MA, Kostov MS, Katic VP: Malignant schwannoma of the pancreas involving transversal colon treated with en-bloc resection. World J Gastroenterol 2010;16:119–122.

16 Coombs RJ: Case of the season. Malignant neurogenic tumor of duodenum and pancreas. Semin Roentgenol 1990;25:127–129.

17 Walsh MM, Brandspigel K: Gastrointestinal bleeding due to pancreatic schwannoma complicating von Recklinghausen's disease. Gastroenterology 1989;97:1550–1551.

18 Eggermont A, Vuzevski V, Huisman M, De Jong K, Jeekel J: Solitary malignant schwannoma of the pancreas: report of a case and ultrastructural examination. J Surg Oncol 1987;36:21–25.

19 Móller Pedersen V, Hede A, Graem N: A solitary malignant schwannoma mimicking a pancreatic pseudocyst. A case report. Acta Chir Scand 1982; 148:697–698.

20 Paranjape C, Johnson SR, Khwaja K, Goldman H, Kruskal JB, Hanto DW: Clinical characteristics, treatment, and outcome of pancreatic Schwannomas. J Gastrointest Surg 2004;8:706–712.

21 Li Q, Gao C, Juzi JT, Hao X: Analysis of 82 cases of retroperitoneal Schwannoma. ANZ J Surg 2007; 77:237–240.

22 Li S, Ai SZ, Owens C, Kulesza P: Intrapancreatic schwannoma diagnosed by endoscopic ultrasound-guided fine-needle aspiration cytology. Diagn Cytopathol 2009;37:132–135.

23 Nakamura Y, Egami K, Maeda S, Hosone M, Onda M: Primary leiomyoma of the pancreas. Int J Pancreatol 2000;28:235–238.

24 Wisniewski B, Vadrot J, Couvelard A: Primary leiomyoma of the head of pancreas. A case report. Gastroenterol Clin Biol 2006;30:137–138.

25 Sato T, Kato S, Watanabe S, Hosono K, Kobayashi N, Nakajima A, Kubota K: Primary leiomyoma of the pancreas diagnosed by endoscopic ultrasound-guided fine-needle aspiration. Dig Endosc 2012;24:380.

26 Søreide JA, Undersrud ES, Al-Saiddi MS, Tholfsen T, Søreide K: Primary leiomyosarcoma of the pancreas – a case report and a comprehensive review. J Gastrointest Cancer 2016;47:358–365.

27 Zhang H, Jensen MH, Farnell MB, Smyrk TC, Zhang L: Primary leiomyosarcoma of the pancreas: study of 9 cases and review of literature. Am J Surg Pathol 2010;34:1849–1856.

28 Reyes MC, Huang X, Bain A, Ylagan L: Primary pancreatic leiomyosarcoma with metastasis to the liver diagnosed by endoscopic ultrasound-guided fine needle aspiration and fine needle biopsy: a case report and review of literature. Diagn Cytopathol 2016;44:1070–1073.

29 Hebert-Magee S, Varadarajulu S, Frost AR, Ramesh J: Primary pancreatic leiomyosarcoma: a rare diagnosis obtained by EUS-FNA cytology. Gastrointest Endosc 2014;80:361–362.

30 Hornick JL, Fletcher CDM: PEComa: what do we know so far? Histopathology 2006;48:75–82.

31 Okuwaki K, Kida M, Masutani H, Yamauchi H, Katagiri H, Mikami T, Miyazawa S, Iwai T, Takezawa M, Imaizumi H, Koizumi W: A resected perivascular epithelioid cell tumor (PEComa) of the pancreas diagnosed using endoscopic ultrasound guided fine-needle aspiration. Intern Med 2013;52:2061–2066.

32 Jiang H, Ta N, Huang XY, Zhang MH, Xu JJ, Zheng KL, Jin G, Zheng JM: Pancreatic perivascular epithelioid cell tumor: a case report with clinicopathological features and a literature review. World J Gastroenterol 2016;22:3693–3700.

33 Tian YT, Liu H, Shi SS, Xie YB, Xu Q, Zhang JW, Zhao DB, Wang CF, Chen YT: Malignant extra-gastrointestinal stromal tumor of the pancreas: report of two cases and review of the literature. World J Gastroenterol 2014;20:863–868.

34 Liu Z, Tian Y, Xu G, Liu S, Guo M, Lian X, Fan D, Zhang H, Feng F: Pancreatic gastrointestinal stromal tumor: clinicopathologic features and prognosis. J Clin Gastroenterol 2017;51:850–856.

35 Rubin BP: Gastrointestinal stromal tumours: an update. Histopathology 2006;48:83–96.

36 Wieczorek TJ, Faquin WC, Rubin BP, Cibas ES: Cytologic diagnosis of gastrointestinal stromal tumor with emphasis on the differential diagnosis with leiomyosarcoma. Cancer 2001;93:276–287.

37 Vij M, Agrawal V, Pandey R: Malignant extra-gastrointestinal stromal tumor of the pancreas. A case report and review of literature. JOP 2011;12:200–204.

38 Pauser U, Kosmahl M, Sipos B, Klöppel G: Mesenchymal tumors of the pancreas. Surprising, but not uncommon. Pathologe 2005;26:52–58.

Dr. Jasreman Dhillon
Moffitt Cancer Center
12902 USF Magnolia Drive
Tampa, FL 33612 (USA)
jasreman.dhillon@moffitt.org

Author Index

Subject Index